Table of contents

SUGARLESS

COOKBOOK

Unlocking Sweet Freedom
A Comprehensive Guide to a
Sugarless Lifestyle with
Delectable 60 Mouthwatering
Recipes and Empowering
Strategies to Conquer Your
Addiction

JESSICA M. STEVEN

INTRODUCTION

In a world where sweetness is often synonymous with pleasure, it's easy to overlook the hidden dangers that sugar poses to our health. Beyond the delightful taste, sugar can insidiously infiltrate our diets, leading to overeating and a host of health issues. In this exploration, we unravel the intricate relationship between sugar consumption, overeating, and its detrimental effects on overall well-being.

The Sweet Seduction: A Culprit in Overeating
1. Immediate Gratification, Long-Term Consequences
At its core, sugar is a quick source of energy that the body readily absorbs. When consumed, it causes a rapid surge in blood sugar levels, leading to an almost instantaneous feeling of euphoria and increased energy. This immediate reward triggers a psychological response that associates sugar with pleasure, making us crave more.

2. Disrupting the Appetite Regulation Mechanism
The human body has a sophisticated system for regulating appetite and signaling fullness. However, excessive sugar intake can disrupt this delicate balance. High sugar levels can desensitize the body to the hormone leptin, which is responsible for signaling fullness. As a result, individuals may find themselves eating more than necessary, chasing the elusive satisfaction that sugar promises.

3. The Vicious Cycle of Sugar and Emotional Eating:
Sugar often becomes a comforting companion during times of stress or emotional turmoil. The release of "feel-good" chemicals, such as serotonin, in response to sugar consumption creates a temporary escape from emotional distress. This association between sugar and emotional relief can lead to a habitual reliance on sugary treats, fostering overeating as a coping mechanism.

The Hidden Perils: Health Implications of Excessive Sugar Consumption
1. Weight Gain and Obesity
The link between sugar and weight gain is well-established. Excessive sugar intake contributes to the accumulation of visceral fat, increasing the risk of obesity. As overeating becomes a consequence of sugar addiction, the caloric surplus further exacerbates the challenge of weight management.

2. Insulin Resistance and Type 2 Diabetes
Prolonged exposure to high sugar levels can lead to insulin resistance, a condition where cells no longer respond effectively to insulin. This disruption in insulin function is a precursor to type 2 diabetes, a chronic health condition with severe implications for overall well-being.

3. Cardiovascular Complications
Overeating, particularly on a diet high in sugar, can contribute to elevated blood pressure and cholesterol levels. These factors, combined with the inflammatory response triggered by excessive sugar consumption, create a perfect storm for cardiovascular complications, including heart disease.

Breaking the Chains: Strategies for a Sugar-Free Lifestyle

Understanding the impact of sugar on overeating and health is the first step toward reclaiming control over our well-being. To break free from the sweet seduction, consider the following strategies:

1. Educate Yourself
Arm yourself with knowledge about hidden sugars in processed foods and understand how they contribute to overeating. Reading food labels can be an eye-opener in recognizing and reducing your sugar intake.

2. Gradual Reduction
Cold-turkey approaches to sugar elimination can be challenging. Instead, opt for a gradual reduction in sugar intake. Replace sugary snacks with healthier alternatives, gradually weaning yourself off excessive sweetness.

3. Embrace Whole Foods
Base your diet on whole, unprocessed foods. Fruits, vegetables, lean proteins, and whole grains can provide the necessary nutrients without the added sugars found in many processed foods.

4. Mindful Eating
Practice mindful eating by paying attention to hunger and fullness cues. Slowing down during meals and savoring each bite can help recalibrate your relationship with food and reduce the tendency to overeat.

In conclusion, understanding how sugar triggers overeating and harms your health is pivotal in making informed choices for a balanced and nourishing lifestyle. By unraveling the sweet menace, you empower yourself to break free from the clutches of excessive sugar consumption, paving the way for improved well-being and long-term health.

Sugar's Stealthy Tactics
Unmasking the Hidden Culprits in Your Everyday Diet

In the quest for a healthier lifestyle, one of the most formidable adversaries is sugar, and it has a knack for hiding in plain sight within our daily diets. Despite our best intentions, sugar sneaks into various foods, often masquerading under innocent-sounding names. In this exploration, we uncover the covert operations of sugar, revealing where it hides and how to navigate the deceptive landscape of hidden sugars.

The Sweet Saboteur: A Closer Look at Hidden Sugars

1. Common Culprits in Disguise

Sugar goes by many aliases, and it's essential to recognize these covert identities on food labels. Ingredients such as sucrose, high fructose corn syrup, agave nectar, and even terms like "evaporated cane juice" can all be sugar in disguise. Understanding these hidden names empowers you to make informed choices when selecting your groceries.

2. The Sneaky Seduction of Processed Foods

Processed foods, often labeled as convenient and time-saving, are notorious for harboring hidden sugars. From seemingly healthy yogurt to savory sauces and condiments, the sugar content in these items can be surprisingly high. Scrutinizing nutrition labels is crucial to unveil the true sugar content and make smarter choices for your health.

3. Beverage Betrayal

Sugary beverages are one of the leading culprits in our daily sugar intake, and they often escape our attention. Sodas, energy drinks, and even seemingly innocent fruit juices can be laden with added sugars. Opting for water, herbal teas, or infused water with natural flavors can help sidestep this sugary trap.

Unveiling Hidden Sugar's Health Impact

1. Weight Management Challenges

The insidious nature of hidden sugars contributes significantly to the global obesity epidemic. Often adding unnecessary calories without providing essential nutrients, hidden sugars can sabotage weight management efforts, leading to unwanted pounds and associated health issues.

2. Increased Risk of Chronic Diseases

Regular consumption of hidden sugars is linked to an increased risk of chronic diseases such as type 2 diabetes and cardiovascular issues. The body's struggle to process excessive sugar can lead to insulin resistance, inflammation, and other metabolic disturbances.

3. Energy Rollercoaster

While the initial surge of energy from hidden sugars may be tempting, it's often short-lived, leading to a subsequent crash. This energy rollercoaster can result in fatigue, mood swings, and cravings for more sugar, perpetuating a cycle that can be challenging to break.

Navigating the Sugar-Laden Landscape: Strategies for a Sugar Savvy Diet

1. Empower Yourself with Label Literacy

Develop the habit of reading nutrition labels diligently. Look out for various names of sugar and choose products with lower sugar content. Consider alternative products or, better yet, prepare fresh meals with whole ingredients whenever possible.

2. Cooking at Home

Taking control of your meals by cooking at home allows you to monitor and regulate the ingredients in your dishes. This not only helps you avoid hidden sugars but also promotes a diet rich in whole, nutrient-dense foods.

3. Choose Whole Foods

Opt for whole, unprocessed foods that are naturally low in added sugars. Fruits, vegetables, lean proteins, and whole grains should form the foundation of your diet, providing essential nutrients without the hidden sugars found in many processed foods.

4. Mindful Consumption

Cultivate a mindful approach to eating by savoring each bite and paying attention to your body's hunger and fullness cues. This mindful consumption not only helps prevent overeating but also allows you to appreciate the natural flavors of whole foods

Craving Sweet Freedom
Unveiling the Addictive Grip of Sugar on the Brain

In the modern world, the allure of sugar is omnipresent, tempting us with its sweet embrace at every turn. Beyond its delectable taste, sugar possesses a dark secret – an addictive nature that can captivate the brain and wreak havoc on our well-being. In this exploration, we delve into the intricate relationship between sugar and the brain, uncovering the mechanisms that make it a potent, albeit stealthy, addiction.

The Sweet Siren's Call: How Sugar Captivates the Brain

1. Dopamine, the Pleasure Messenger
At the heart of sugar's addictive nature lies its profound impact on the brain's reward system. Consumption of sugar triggers the release of dopamine, a neurotransmitter associated with pleasure and reward. This surge creates a euphoric sensation, imprinting a positive association between sugar intake and feeling good.

2. The Brain's Response to Sugar Binges
With repeated exposure, the brain adapts by reducing the sensitivity of its reward system. This desensitization prompts individuals to seek higher quantities or more intense forms of sugar to achieve the same pleasurable effect, setting the stage for overconsumption and potential addiction.

3. Cravings, Habits, and Rituals
Sugar not only alters the brain's reward system but also ingrains itself in our habits and daily rituals. The brain forms strong neural connections associated with sugar consumption, leading to cravings and a seemingly automatic response to stress or emotional triggers.

Unraveling the Impact
How Sugar Addiction Affects Mental and Physical Health

1. Emotional Rollercoaster
The highs and lows associated with sugar-induced dopamine spikes create an emotional rollercoaster. The temporary euphoria followed by the inevitable crash can contribute to mood swings, irritability, and an increased susceptibility to stress.

2. Physical Consequences
Beyond its impact on mental health, sugar addiction takes a toll on the body. Excessive sugar consumption is linked to inflammation, insulin resistance, and an increased risk of chronic diseases, including obesity, type 2 diabetes, and cardiovascular issues.

3. The Cycle of Dependency
Sugar addiction perpetuates a cycle of dependency, where cravings lead to consumption, and consumption reinforces cravings. Breaking free from this cycle requires a concerted effort to address both the physical and psychological aspects of addiction.

Breaking the Sweet Shackles: Strategies for Overcoming Sugar Addiction

1. Mindful Consumption
Practicing mindful eating involves paying attention to the sensations of hunger and fullness, savoring each bite, and being aware of the emotions that may trigger sugar cravings. This mindful approach helps break automatic responses to sugar stimuli.

2. Gradual Reduction
Abruptly cutting out all sugar can be challenging and lead to withdrawal symptoms. A more sustainable approach involves gradual reduction, replacing sugary snacks with healthier alternatives, and allowing the taste buds to adjust over time.

3. Balanced Diet and Hydration
A well-balanced diet that includes whole foods and proper hydration can help stabilize blood sugar levels and reduce the intensity of sugar cravings. Ensuring adequate nutrient intake supports overall health and reduces the reliance on sugary treats.

4. Seeking Support
Overcoming sugar addiction is a journey that can benefit from support. Whether through friends, family, or professional guidance, seeking support provides encouragement, accountability, and a sense of community in the quest for sugar-free living.

The Path to Sweet Freedom: Embracing a Healthier Relationship with Sugar

Breaking Sweet Chains
Practical Steps to Embrace a Sugarless Lifestyle

In a world where sugar-laden temptations lurk around every corner, breaking free from the clutches of sugar dependence is a courageous journey towards improved health and vitality. As we embark on the path to a sugarless lifestyle, it's crucial to equip ourselves with practical strategies that empower lasting change. In this guide, we'll explore actionable steps to liberate ourselves from sugar's hold and embrace a lifestyle that fosters well-being.

Understanding the Foundations
The Why and How of Sugar Dependence

1. Educate Yourself

Knowledge is power, and understanding the impact of sugar on your health is the first step to breaking dependence. Research the effects of sugar on the body, from its contribution to weight gain and inflammation to its role in chronic diseases. This awareness forms the bedrock of your commitment to change.

2. Audit Your Current Sugar Intake

Take stock of your daily diet to identify hidden sources of sugar. Scrutinize food labels and be mindful of seemingly innocent culprits like condiments, sauces, and processed snacks. Awareness of your current sugar intake provides a clear starting point for making informed decisions.

3. Set Clear and Realistic Goals

Establish specific, measurable, and achievable goals for reducing sugar in your diet. Whether it's cutting out sugary beverages, minimizing desserts, or opting for healthier snack alternatives, setting clear goals provides a roadmap for success.

Practical Strategies for a Sugarless Lifestyle

1. Reformulate Your Plate

Center your meals around whole, nutrient-dense foods. Incorporate a variety of colorful fruits, vegetables, lean proteins, and whole grains. This not only reduces reliance on processed foods but also ensures a balanced intake of essential nutrients.

2. Sugar Swap

Replace refined sugars with natural sweeteners like honey, maple syrup, or stevia in your recipes. Gradually decrease the amount of sweetener used to allow your taste buds to adjust. Experiment with herbs and spices to add flavor without the need for excessive sweetness.

3. Meal Preparation and Planning

Taking control of your food preparation allows you to monitor and regulate the ingredients in your meals. Set aside time for weekly meal planning and prep to ensure you have nourishing, sugar-free options readily available.

4. Stay Hydrated

Thirst is often mistaken for hunger, leading to unnecessary snacking. Stay hydrated by drinking plenty of water throughout the day. Infuse your water with citrus slices, berries, or mint for a refreshing and naturally flavored alternative.

5. Mindful Eating Practices

Cultivate mindfulness during meals by savoring each bite, chewing slowly, and paying attention to hunger and fullness cues. Engaging your senses in the act of eating enhances your appreciation for the flavors of whole foods and reduces the desire for added sweetness.

Coping with Challenges Strategies for Long-Term Success

1. Build a Support System
Share your journey with friends, family, or a support group. Having a network of encouragement provides accountability, motivation, and a sense of community in the face of challenges.

2. Celebrate Small Wins
Acknowledge and celebrate your achievements along the way. Whether it's resisting a sugary temptation or successfully incorporating a new sugarless recipe, recognizing small wins reinforces your commitment to a sugarless lifestyle.

3. Learn from Setbacks
Acknowledge that setbacks may occur, and use them as opportunities to learn and grow. Analyze the circumstances surrounding a lapse in your sugarless journey and strategize how to overcome similar challenges in the future.

Navigating the Sugar Maze Effective Coping Mechanisms for Reducing Sugar Consumption

Embarking on a journey to reduce sugar consumption is a commendable commitment to one's health and well-being. However, the path to a sugarless lifestyle is not without its challenges. From cravings to social pressures, various hurdles can make this transition seem daunting. In this comprehensive guide, we explore practical coping mechanisms to empower you in handling the hurdles and achieving success on your journey to significantly reduce sugar consumption.

Identifying and Addressing Sugar Cravings

1. Understand the Source

Cravings often signal a deeper need or emotion. Identifying the root cause of your sugar cravings—whether it's stress, boredom, or habit—allows you to address the underlying issue rather than succumb to the craving.

2. Satisfy with Alternatives

Instead of completely denying your sweet tooth, satisfy it with healthier alternatives. Fresh fruits, naturally sweetened snacks, or homemade treats using minimal sweeteners can help curb cravings while keeping your sugar intake in check.

3. Hydration as a Craving Buster

Often, dehydration can be mistaken for hunger or cravings. Keep hydrated throughout the day by drinking water or herbal teas, as staying well-hydrated can help reduce the intensity of sugar cravings.

Navigating Social Pressures and Gatherings

1. Communicate Your Goals
Open communication is key. Share your commitment to reducing sugar consumption with friends and family. This not only sets expectations but also invites support and understanding, making social situations more conducive to your goals.

2. Bring Your Own
When attending gatherings or events, bring your own sugar-free dishes or snacks. This ensures you have satisfying options that align with your goals and helps overcome the temptation of indulging in sugary offerings.

3. Learn to Say No Gracefully
Politeness can sometimes lead to succumbing to peer pressure. Practice saying no gracefully and with confidence. Remember, your health is a priority, and those who care about you will respect your choices.

Coping with Emotional Eating Triggers

1. Mindful Eating Practices
Adopting mindful eating practices involves paying attention to the sensory experience of eating and being present in the moment. This can help break the cycle of emotional eating and promote a healthier relationship with food.

2. Alternative Coping Mechanisms
Identify alternative coping mechanisms for stress or emotional distress that do not involve turning to sugary comfort foods. Activities such as deep breathing, exercise, or engaging in hobbies can serve as effective alternatives.

3. Seek Professional Support
If emotional eating is a persistent challenge, consider seeking support from a mental health professional or a nutritionist. They can provide tailored strategies to address emotional triggers and develop a healthier relationship with food.

Overcoming Setbacks and Staying Resilient

1. Embrace Imperfection

Acknowledge that setbacks are a natural part of any transformative journey. Instead of viewing them as failures, consider them learning opportunities. Embrace imperfection, learn from the experience, and recommit to your goals.

2. Focus on Progress, Not Perfection

Celebrate the progress you make, no matter how small. Shifting the focus from achieving perfection to acknowledging continuous improvement fosters a positive mindset and helps maintain motivation.

3. Reevaluate and Adjust Goals

Periodically reassess your goals and make adjustments as needed. Life is dynamic, and your circumstances may change. Flexibility in your approach ensures that your goals remain realistic and achievable.

Sweet Success
Navigating the Three S's in Your Sugar-Reduction Journey
Embarking on a journey to reduce sugar consumption is not just a change in diet; it's a transformative lifestyle shift. However, the road to a sugar-free existence is often laden with stressors, setbacks, and social pressures. In this guide, we delve into strategies to effectively navigate the three S's—stressors, setbacks, and social pressures enabling you to stay resilient and successful in your quest to reduce sugar consumption.

Managing Stressors
Finding Calm Amidst the Chaos

1. Incorporate Stress-Reducing Activities
Stress can be a significant trigger for sugar cravings. Integrate stress-reducing activities into your routine, such as meditation, yoga, or deep breathing exercises. These practices not only alleviate stress but also provide healthier alternatives to cope with daily pressures.

2. Prioritize Self-Care
Ensure you are prioritizing self-care in your daily life. Adequate sleep, regular exercise, and moments of relaxation contribute to overall well-being, reducing the likelihood of succumbing to stress-induced sugar cravings.

3. Establish Healthy Boundaries
Learn to recognize and set boundaries in your personal and professional life. Establishing clear boundaries helps minimize stressors and allows you to focus on your sugar-reduction goals without unnecessary distractions.

Overcoming Setbacks
Turning Challenges into Opportunities

1. Cultivate a Growth Mindset
View setbacks as opportunities for growth rather than failures. A growth mindset allows you to learn from challenges, adjust your approach, and strengthen your resolve to move forward on your sugar-reduction journey.

2. Learn from Mistakes
Analyze the circumstances surrounding setbacks without self-judgment. Identify triggers, situations, or emotions that led to the setback, and use this knowledge to implement proactive strategies for future success.

3. Reassess and Adjust Goals
Periodically reassess your sugar-reduction goals. If setbacks become recurring, consider adjusting your goals to ensure they are realistic and attainable, setting the stage for consistent progress.

Navigating Social Pressures, Staying True to Your Goals

1. Communicate Your Choices
Transparent communication is essential. Articulate your commitment to reducing sugar to friends and family, explaining the health motivations behind your decision. This fosters understanding and diminishes social pressures to conform.

2. Lead by Example
Demonstrate the benefits of a sugar-reduced lifestyle by being an example. Share your experiences, the positive changes you've noticed, and your favorite sugar-free recipes. Leading by example can inspire others and diminish external pressures.

3. Bring Your Own
When attending social gatherings, contribute sugar-free dishes or snacks to ensure there are options aligning with your goals. Bringing your own treats not only guarantees healthier alternatives but also showcases the delicious possibilities of a sugar-free lifestyle.

Building Resilience for Long-Term Success

1. Cultivate a Support System
Surround yourself with a supportive network. Share your goals
with friends, family, or join online communities dedicated to a
sugar-free lifestyle. Having a support system provides
encouragement and understanding during challenging times.

2. Celebrate Non-Scale Victories
Acknowledge and celebrate victories beyond the scale.
Recognize improvements in energy levels, mood, and overall
well-being. Celebrating non-scale victories reinforces the
positive impact of your sugar-reduction efforts.

3. Mindful Reflection
Regularly reflect on your journey. Consider keeping a journal to
track progress, challenges, and your emotional state. Mindful
reflection enhances self-awareness and equips you with valuable
insights for continued success.

Sugarless for Life
Nurturing Long-Term Success in Embracing a Sugar
Free Lifestyle

Embarking on the journey to a sugar-free lifestyle is a commendable decision that promises a host of benefits for both physical and mental well-being. However, the key to true success lies not just in adopting this lifestyle momentarily but in sustaining it for the long term. In this guide, we delve into the strategies and mindset shifts that will help you nurture long-term success in embracing a sugar-free lifestyle.

Cultivating a Mindset Shift
From Restriction to Empowerment

1. Focus on Abundance, Not Deprivation
Shift your perspective from what you are giving up to what you are gaining. Embrace the abundance of nutrient-dense, whole foods that form the foundation of a sugar-free lifestyle. Celebrate the variety and flavors these foods offer, making the journey an exploration of culinary richness.

2. View It as a Lifestyle, Not a Diet
Avoid thinking of your sugar-free journey as a temporary diet. Instead, perceive it as a sustainable lifestyle change. Diets often come with an expiration date, while a lifestyle shift is an enduring commitment to your health and well-being.

3. Embrace Flexibility
Recognize that perfection is not the goal. Allow yourself flexibility and occasional indulgences without guilt. This approach fosters a healthier relationship with food, reducing the chances of feeling restricted and increasing the likelihood of long-term success.

Building a Sustainable Meal Plan

1. Diversify Your Plate

Keep your meals exciting and nutrient-packed by incorporating a diverse range of fruits, vegetables, lean proteins, and whole grains. Experiment with different cooking techniques and flavor combinations to ensure a rich and satisfying culinary experience.

2. Meal Prep for Convenience

Simplify your sugar-free lifestyle by incorporating meal prep into your routine. Preparing meals in advance not only saves time but also ensures that you have convenient, healthy options readily available, reducing the temptation to turn to sugary convenience foods.

3. Discover Sugar-Free Alternatives

Explore and integrate sugar-free alternatives into your recipes. Natural sweeteners like stevia, monk fruit, or erythritol can be excellent substitutes. Experiment with these alternatives to find what suits your taste buds while keeping your sugar intake minimal.

Mindful Eating Practices

1. Eat with Intention

Mindful eating involves being fully present during meals, savoring each bite, and paying attention to hunger and fullness cues. Eating with intention enhances the enjoyment of your food and promotes a balanced relationship with nourishment.

2. Listen to Your Body

Learn to discern between physical hunger and emotional cravings. Listening to your body's signals and responding appropriately helps foster a sustainable, intuitive approach to eating, reducing the likelihood of overindulgence in sugary treats.

3. Chew Slowly and Enjoy the Experience

Slow down during meals, chew your food thoroughly, and relish the experience. Not only does this promote better digestion, but it also allows you to appreciate the natural flavors of your meals, reducing the desire for added sweetness.

Establishing a Supportive Environmen

1. Communicate Your Goals
Share your sugar-free journey with friends and family. Clear communication helps set expectations and fosters a supportive environment where your loved ones can champion your efforts rather than inadvertently becoming obstacles.
2. Join a Community
Consider joining a community or online group dedicated to a sugar-free lifestyle. Connecting with like-minded individuals provides encouragement, shared experiences, and a sense of community that can be invaluable on the journey to long-term success.
3. Celebrate Milestones
Acknowledge and celebrate milestones in your sugar-free journey. Whether it's a week, a month, or a year without added sugars, recognizing and celebrating achievements reinforces the positive impact of your commitment.

Reflecting on Your Sugar-Free Journey

1. Periodic Self-Reflection
Regularly reflect on your sugar-free journey. Assess your progress, challenges, and how your body and mind have responded to the lifestyle shift. This self-awareness enhances your ability to make informed choices and adjust your approach as needed.
2. Adjust and Evolve
Understand that your sugar-free journey is dynamic. As your circumstances, preferences, and health goals evolve, be open to adjusting your approach. Flexibility and adaptability ensure that your sugar-free lifestyle remains relevant and sustainable over the long term.
3. Set New Challenges
Keep the journey exciting by setting new challenges or goals related to your sugar-free lifestyle. This could involve experimenting with new recipes, exploring different cuisines, or gradually reducing reliance on sugar substitutes. Continual growth and evolution contribute to sustained success.

Beverages

These sugarless beverages offer a spectrum of flavors and health benefits, proving that enjoying delicious drinks doesn't require added sugars. Incorporate these refreshing recipes into your daily routine for a hydrating, flavorful, and health-conscious beverage experience.

Citrus Mint Sparkler

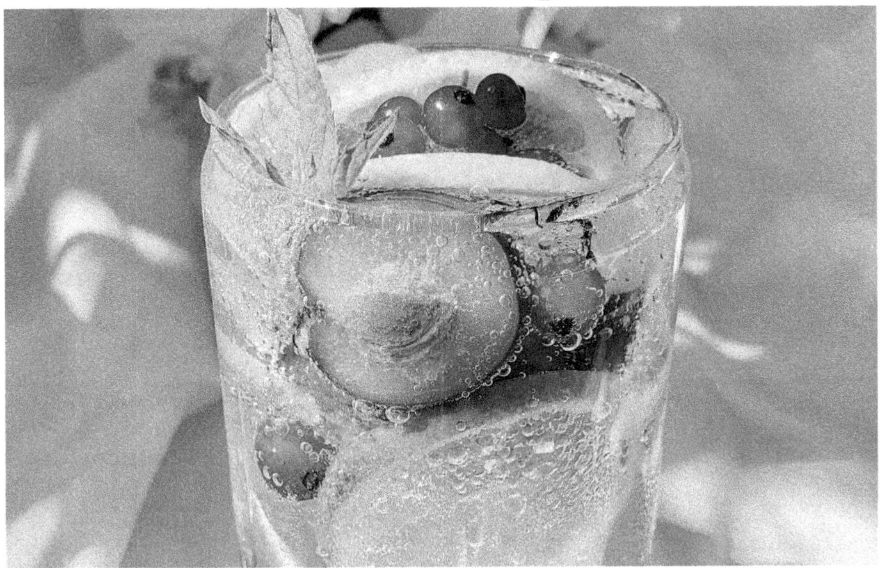

Ingredients

- 2 cups sparkling water
- 1 lime, sliced
- 1 lemon, sliced
- Fresh mint leaves

Nutritional Value

Calories: 0,
Sugar: 0g,
Vitamin C: High, Mint:
Adds freshness and aids digestion.

Instructions

1. Fill two glasses with ice.
2. Squeeze lime and lemon slices into the glasses.
3. Add fresh mint leaves.
4. Pour sparkling water over the ingredients.
5. Stir gently and enjoy!

Brief Description/Backstory

A refreshing blend of citrus and mint, this sparkling beverage is a perfect sugarless pick-me-up on a warm day.

Cucumber Basil Infusion

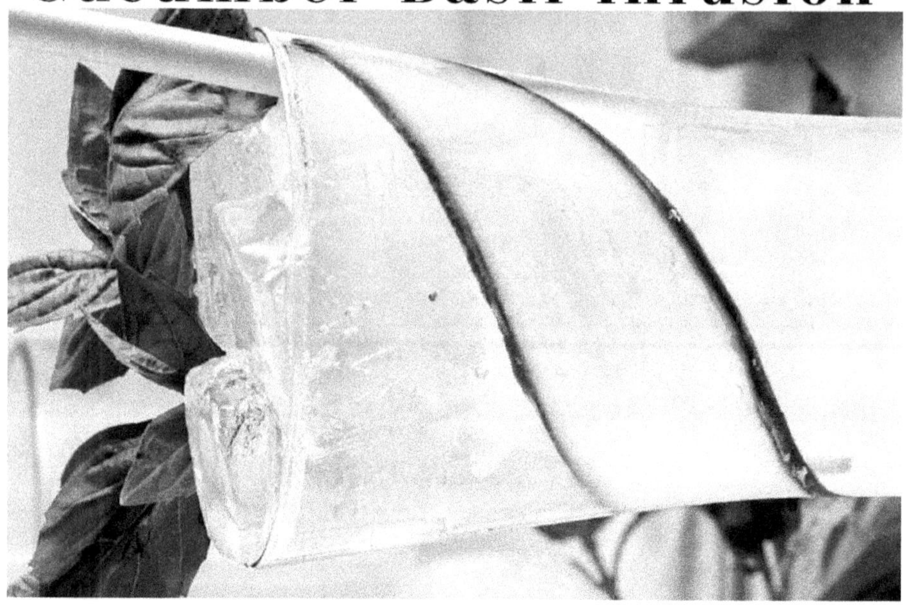

Ingredients

- 1 cucumber, thinly sliced
- Handful of fresh basil leaves
  4 cups water
- Ice cubes

Instructions

1. Place cucumber slices and basil leaves in a pitcher.
2. Add water and refrigerate for at least 2 hours.
3. Pour over ice and savor the refreshing blend.

Nutritional Value

Calories: 0,
Sugar: 0g,
Hydration: High,
Basil: Contains antioxidants.

Brief Description/Backstory

An invigorating sugarless beverage that combines the crispness of cucumber with the aromatic touch of basil, creating a hydrating sensation.

Berry Blast Smoothie

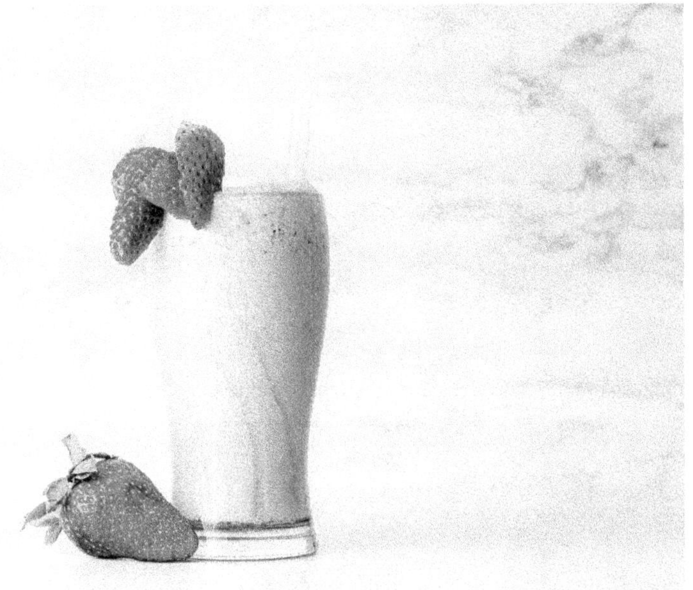

Ingredients

- 1 cup mixed berries (strawberries, blueberries, raspberries)
- 1 cup unsweetened almond milk
- 1 tablespoon chia seeds
- Ice cubes

Instructions

1. Blend mixed berries and almond milk until smooth.
2. Add chia seeds and blend again.
3. Pour over ice and enjoy the berry blast!

Nutritional Value

Calories: 70,
Sugar: 0g,
Fiber: 7g,
Antioxidants: High

Brief Description/Backstory

A vibrant and nutritious smoothie that packs the goodness of mixed berries without any added sugars.

Ginger-Lemon Iced Tea

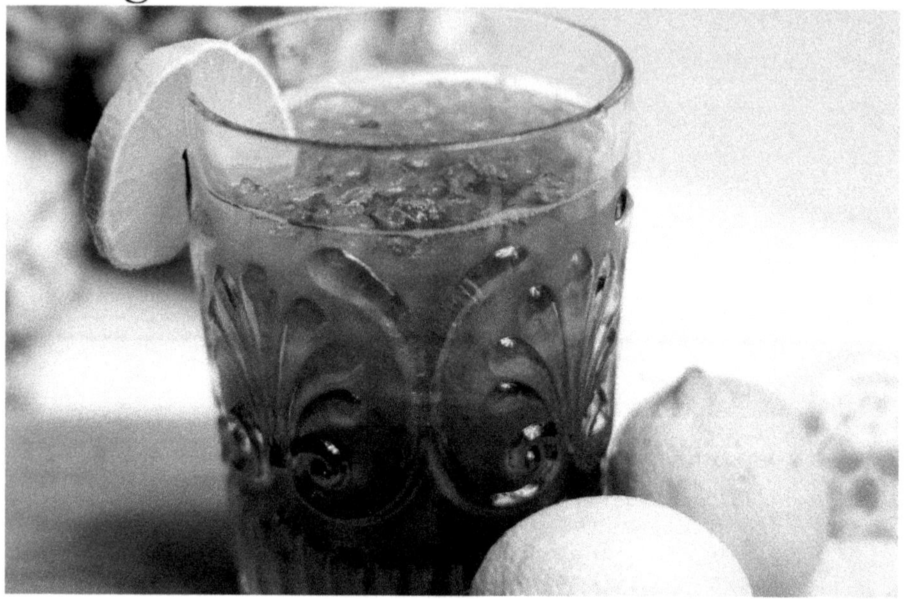

Ingredients

- 2 black tea bags
- 1 tablespoon fresh ginger, grated
- 1 lemon, sliced
- 4 cups water
- Ice cubes

Instructions

1. Brew black tea bags and grated ginger in hot water.
2. Let it cool, then refrigerate.
3. Serve over ice with lemon slices.

Nutritional Value

Calories: 0,
Sugar: 0g,
Ginger: Aids digestion,
Vitamin C: Boosts immunity.

Brief Description/Backstory

A zesty and invigorating iced tea with the warmth of ginger and the citrusy kick of lemon, perfect for a summer day

Pineapple-Mint Cooler

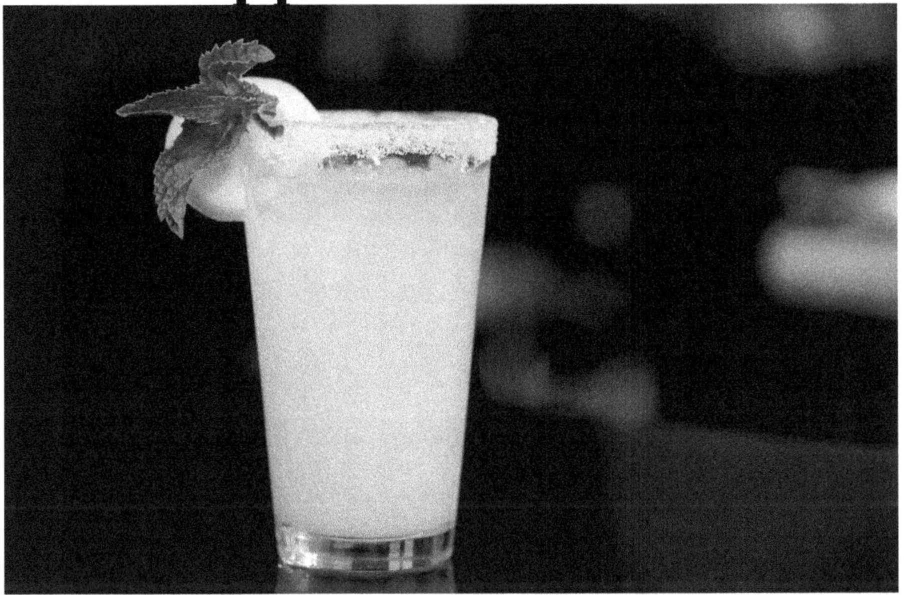

Ingredients

- 1 cup fresh pineapple chunks
- Handful of fresh mint leaves
- 2 cups coconut water
- Ice cubes

Instructions

1. Blend pineapple chunks and mint leaves with coconut water.
2. Strain the mixture for a smoother texture.
3. Serve over ice and enjoy the tropical refreshment.

Nutritional Value

Calories: 100,
Sugar: 0g,
Vitamin C: High,
Electrolytes: Coconut water hydrates.

Brief Description/Backstory

A tropical delight that combines the sweetness of pineapple with the freshness of mint, creating a delightful and sugarless cooler.

Green Apple Cinnamon Detox Water

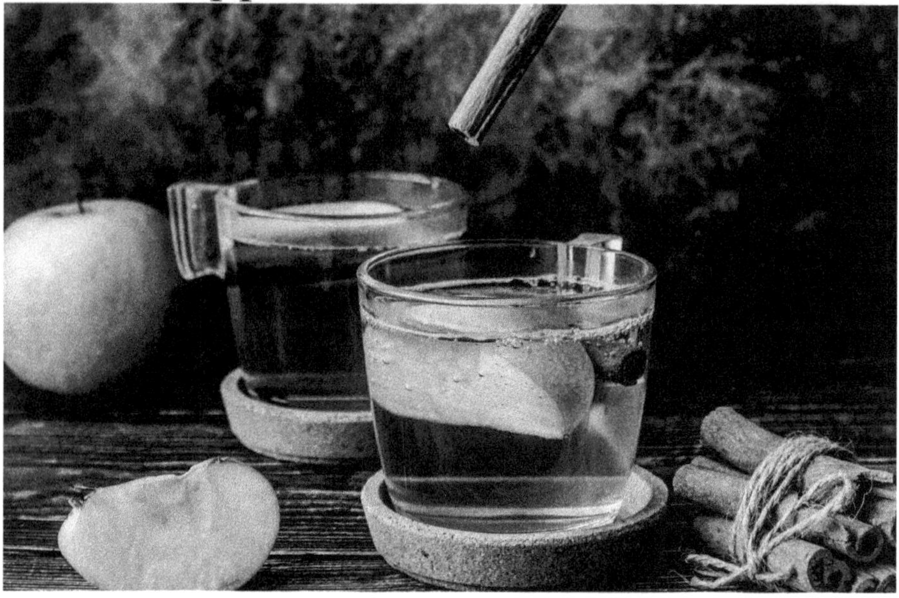

Ingredients

- 1 green apple, thinly sliced
- 1 cinnamon stick
- 4 cups water
- Ice cubes

Instructions

1. Combine green apple slices and cinnamon stick in a pitcher.
2. Add water and refrigerate for at least 1 hour.
3. Pour over ice and experience a refreshing detox.

Nutritional Value

Calories: 50,
Sugar: 0g,
Detoxifying: Cinnamon supports metabolism.

Brief Description/Backstory

A detoxifying beverage that pairs the crispness of green apples with the subtle warmth of cinnamon, promoting hydration.

Herbal Lemonade

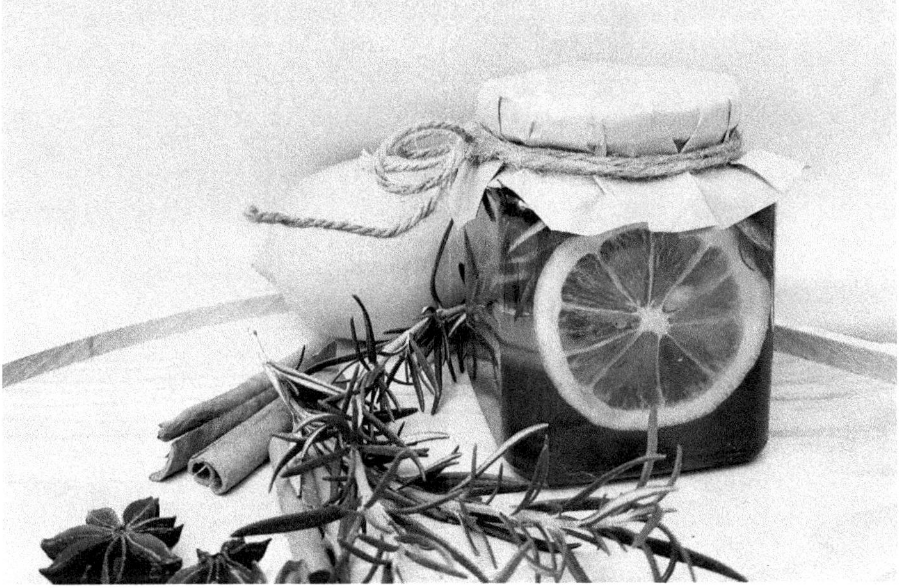

Ingredients

- 2 lemons, juiced
- Handful of fresh herbs (rosemary, thyme, or basil)
- 4 cups water
- Ice cubes

Instructions

1. Mix lemon juice and fresh herbs in a pitcher.
2. Add water and let it infuse for 1-2 hours.
3. Strain and serve over ice.

Nutritional Value

Calories: 10,
Sugar: 0g,
Vitamin C: Boosts immunity,
Herbs: Add antioxidants.

Brief Description/Backstory

An herbal twist to classic lemonade, this sugarless beverage combines the tanginess of lemons with the earthiness

Mango-Mint Refresher

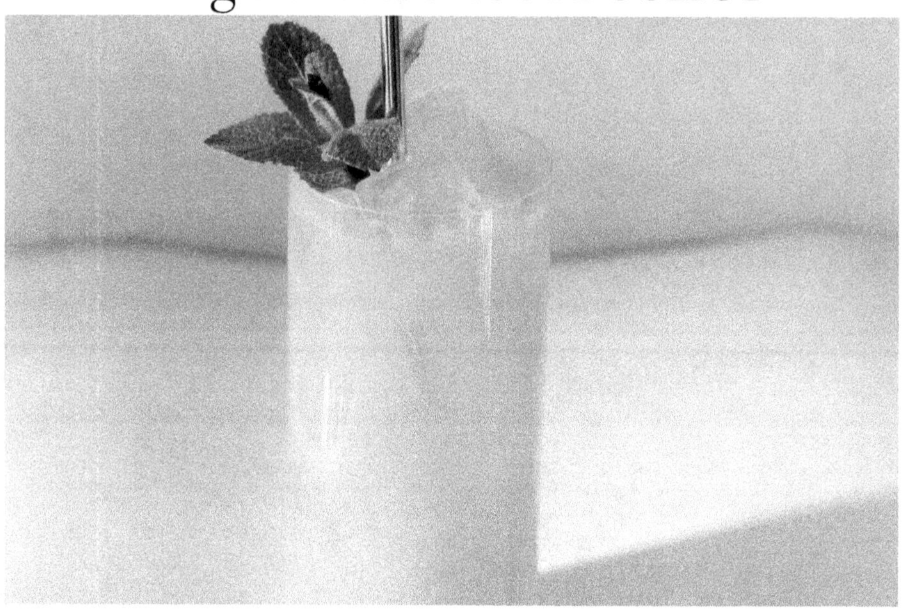

Ingredients

- 1 cup ripe mango chunks
- Handful of fresh mint leaves
- 2 cups water
- Ice cubes

Instructions

1. Blend mango chunks and mint leaves with water.
2. Strain for a smoother consistency.
3. Serve over ice and savor the mango-mint delight.

Nutritional Value

Calories: 80,
Sugar: 0g,
Vitamin A: High,
Mint: Aids digestion.

Brief Description/Backstory

A tropical and rejuvenating beverage that combines the sweetness of mango with the invigorating touch of fresh mint.

Turmeric-Ginger Golden Milk Latte

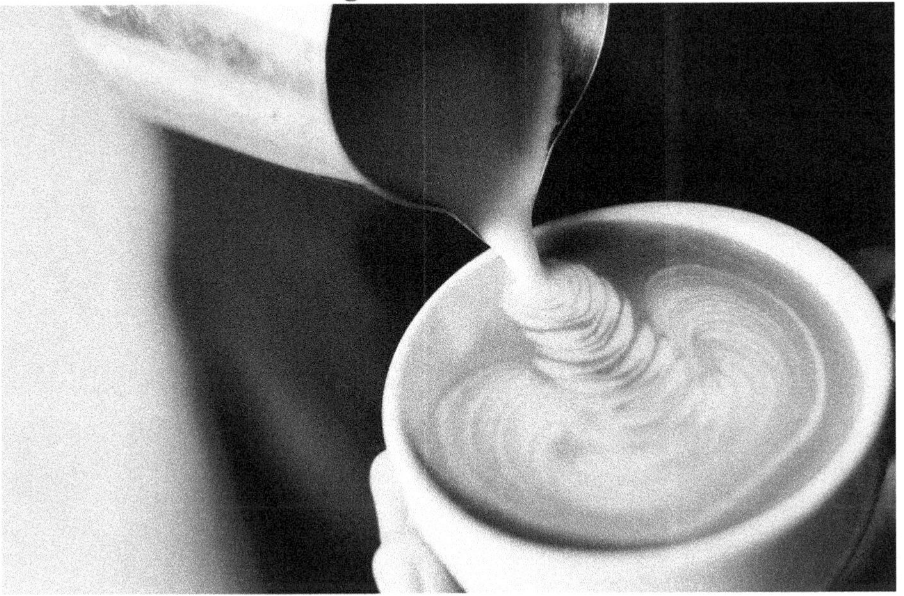

Ingredients

- 2 cups unsweetened almond milk
- 1 teaspoon ground turmeric
- 1 teaspoon fresh ginger, grated
- Pinch of black pepper
- Pinch of cinnamon

Instructions

1. Heat almond milk, turmeric, and ginger in a saucepan.
2. Add black pepper and cinnamon.
3. Whisk until frothy and pour into mugs.

Nutritional Value

Calories: 60,
Sugar: 0g,
Anti-inflammatory:
Turmeric and ginger.

Brief Description/Backstory

A warm and comforting beverage, this golden milk latte combines the anti-inflammatory benefits of turmeric with the spiciness of ginger.

Pomegranate-Basil Spritzer

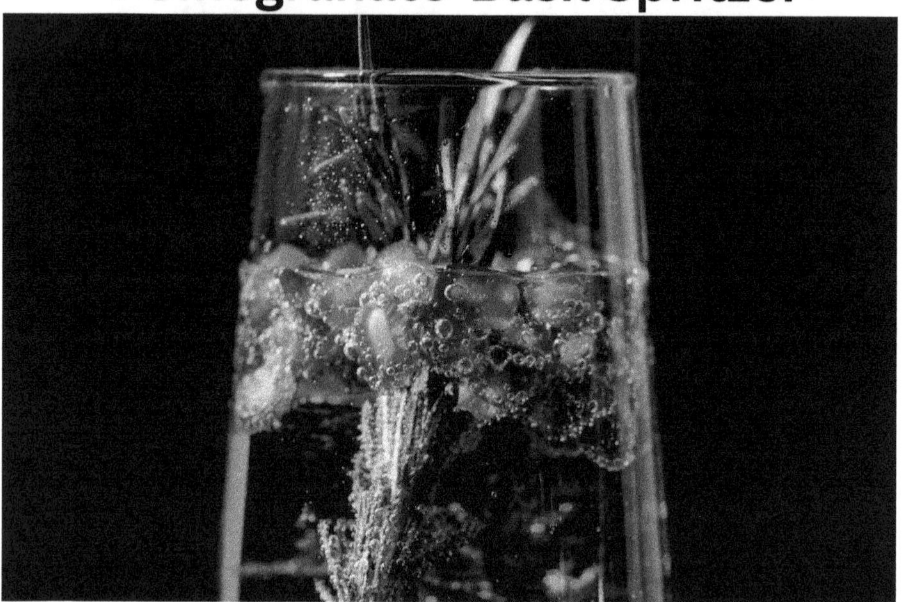

Ingredients

- cup pomegranate seeds
- Handful of fresh basil leaves
- 2 cups sparkling water
- Ice cubes

Instructions

1. Muddle pomegranate seeds and basil leaves in a glass.
2. Fill the glass with ice and pour sparkling water over the mixture.
3. Stir gently and enjoy the vibrant spritzer.

Nutritional Value

Calories: 50,
Sugar: 0g,
Antioxidants: High,
Basil: Adds freshness.

Brief Description/Backstory

A delightful spritzer that combines the tartness of pomegranate with the aromatic notes of fresh basil, creating a unique and sugarless beverage.

Breakfast

These sugarless breakfast delights are not only delicious but also packed with nutrients to fuel your day. From savory omelettes to sweet chia seed puddings, these recipes offer a variety of options to keep your breakfasts both wholesome and satisfying. Enjoy the flavors and benefits of these nutritious morning meals!

Quinoa and Berry Breakfast Bowl

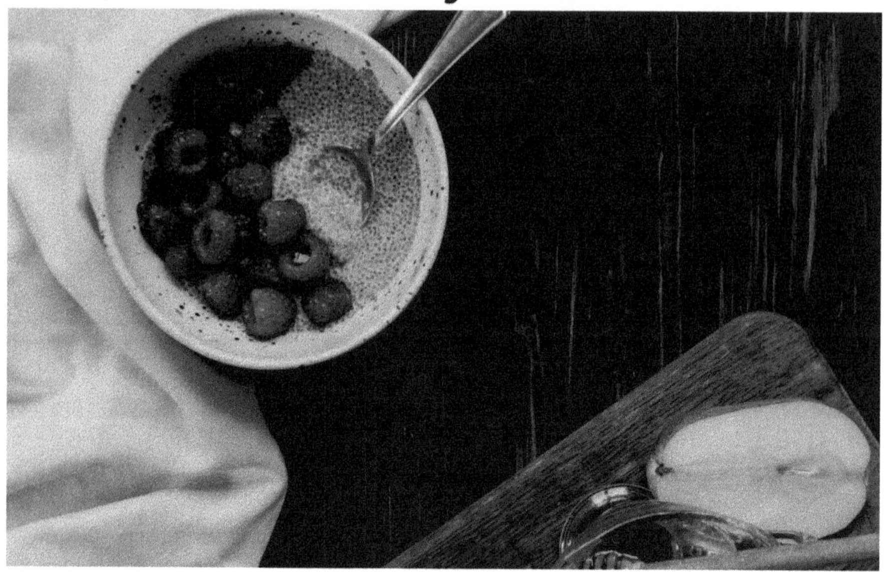

Ingredients

- 1 cup cooked quinoa
- 1 cup mixed berries (strawberries, blueberries, raspberries)
- 1 tablespoon chia seeds
- 2 tablespoons unsweetened Greek yogurt
- Drizzle of honey

Instructions

1. Divide cooked quinoa into two bowls.
2. Top with mixed berries, chia seeds, and Greek yogurt.
3. Drizzle with honey if desired.
4. Mix and enjoy

Nutritional Value

Calories: 300,
Protein: 15g,
Fiber: 8g,
Antioxidants: High.

Brief Description/Backstory

A wholesome and protein-packed breakfast bowl featuring quinoa and a medley of fresh berries to kickstart your day with energy and nutrition.

Avocado and Egg Breakfast Wrap

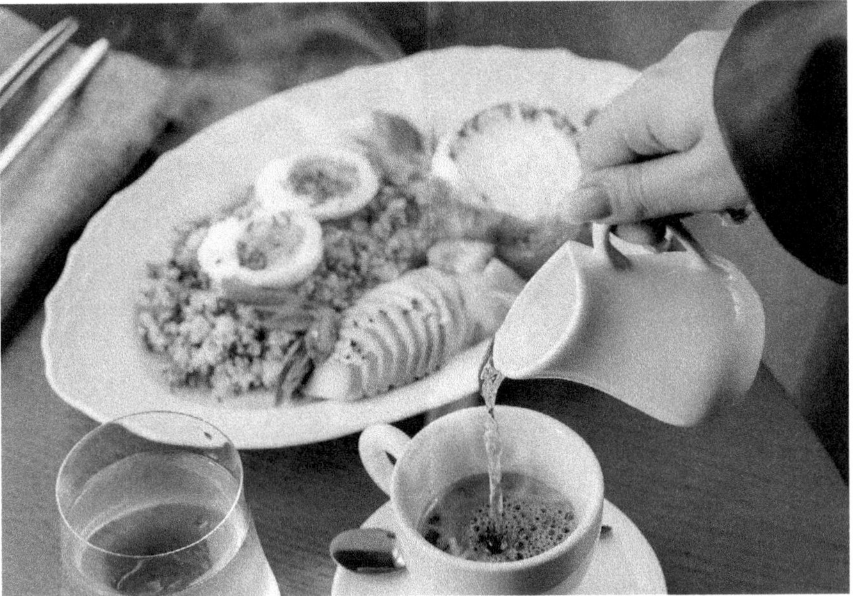

Ingredients

- 2 whole-grain tortillas
- 2 ripe avocados, sliced
- 4 eggs, scrambled
- Salsa for topping
- Salt and pepper to taste

Instructions

1. Warm tortillas in a dry skillet.
2. Layer with sliced avocado and scrambled eggs.
3. Season with salt and pepper.
4. Top with salsa, wrap, and enjoy your hearty breakfast!

Nutritional Value

Calories: 350,
Protein: 14g,
Healthy Fats:
Avocado provides
monounsaturated fats.

Brief Description/Backstory

A savory and satisfying breakfast wrap featuring creamy avocado, protein-rich eggs, and a hint of spice for a perfect morning fuel.

Greek Yogurt Parfait with Granola and Berries

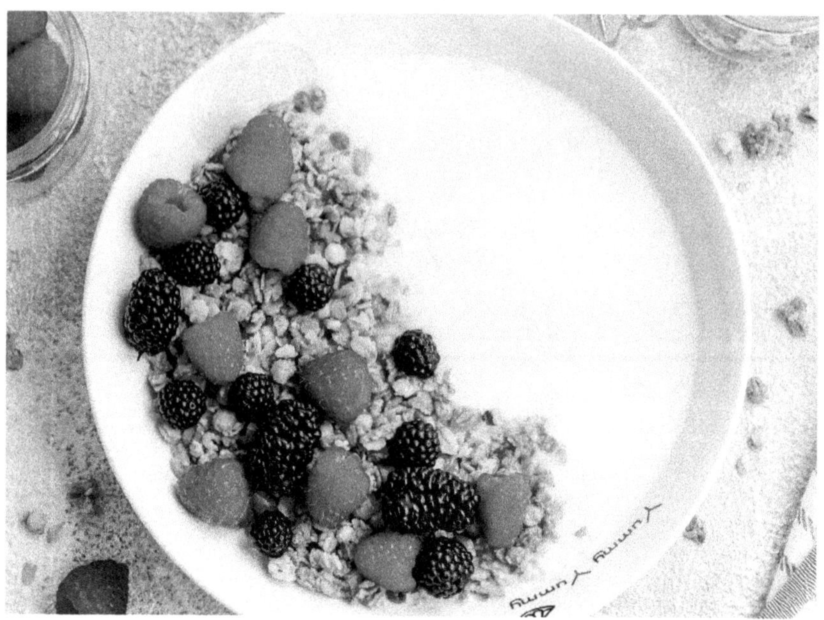

Ingredients

- 2 cups Greek yogurt
- 1 cup granola (sugar-free)
- 1 cup mixed berries
- Drizzle of agave syrup (optional)

Instructions

1. In glasses or bowls, layer Greek yogurt, granola, and mixed berries.
2. Repeat layers.
3. Drizzle with agave syrup if desired.
4. Delight in the parfait of textures and flavors.

Nutritional Value

Calories: 320,
Protein: 20g,
Fiber: 6g,
Probiotics: Greek yogurt promotes gut health.

Brief Description/Backstory

A delightful Greek yogurt parfait layered with crunchy granola and a burst of fresh berries for a balanced and satisfying breakfast.

Sweet Potato and Spinach Breakfast Hash

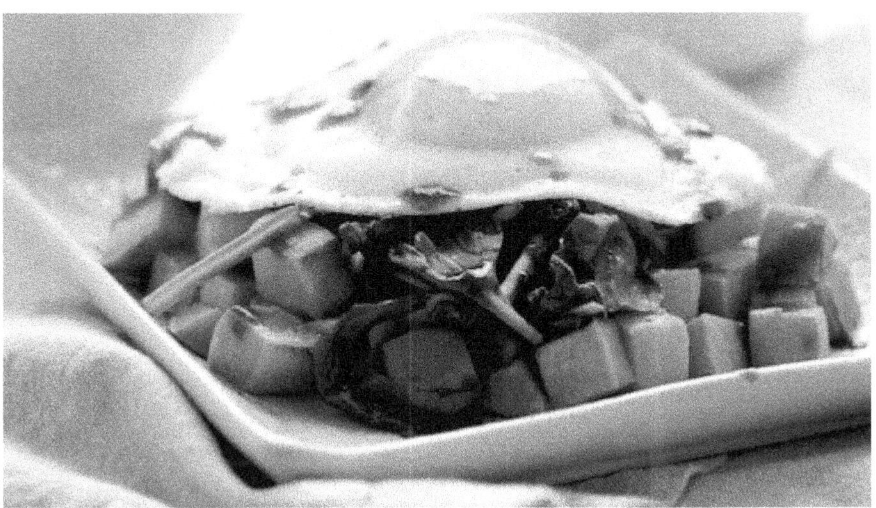

Ingredients

- 2 medium sweet potatoes, diced
- 2 cups fresh spinach
- 1 onion, diced
- 4 eggs
- Olive oil for cooking
- Salt, pepper, and paprika to taste

Instructions

1. Sauté diced sweet potatoes and onions in olive oil until tender.
2. Add fresh spinach and cook until wilted.
3. Season with salt, pepper, and paprika.
4. Create wells in the hash and crack eggs into them.
5. Cover and cook until eggs are done to your liking.

Nutritional Value

Calories: 320,
Protein: 15g,
Vitamin A: High,
Fiber: 7g.

Brief Description/Backstory

A savory breakfast hash featuring nutrient-rich sweet potatoes, sautéed spinach, and a hint of spices for a satisfying and wholesome morning meal.

Chia Seed Pudding with Almond Milk and Berries

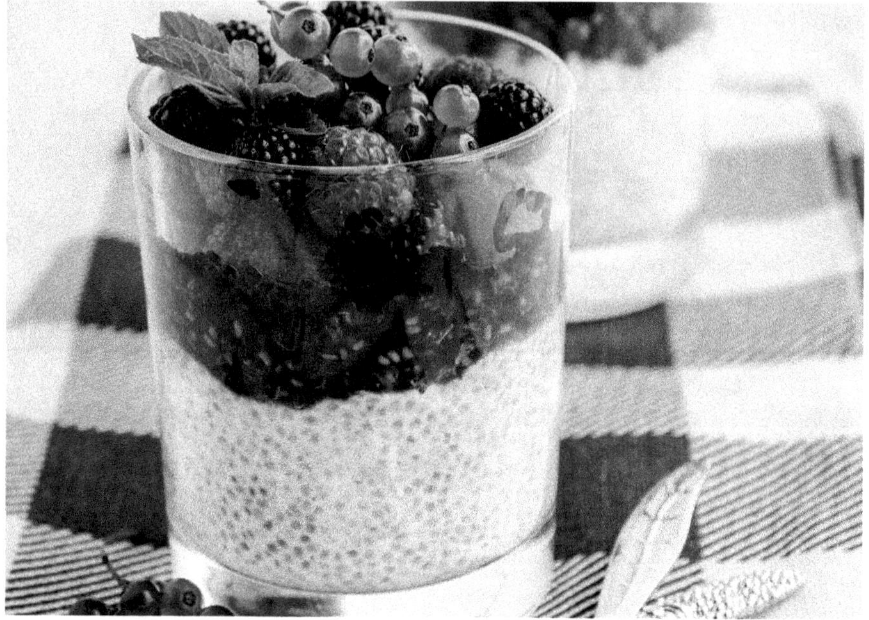

Ingredients

- 1/2 cup chia seeds
- 2 cups unsweetened almond milk
- 1 teaspoon vanilla extract
- 1 cup mixed berries
- Drizzle of maple syrup (optional)

Instructions

1. Mix chia seeds, almond milk, and vanilla extract in a bowl.
2. Refrigerate overnight.
3. In the morning, top with mixed berries.
4. Drizzle with maple syrup if desired.
5. Indulge in a nutritious chia seed pudding.

Nutritional Value

Calories: 250,
Fiber: 15g,
Omega-3 Fatty Acids: Chia seeds are rich in omega-3s.

Brief Description/Backstory

A delightful chia seed pudding made with almond milk and topped with a colorful array of fresh berries, creating a nutritious and visually appealing breakfast.

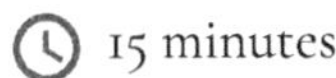

Egg White Omelette with Vegetables

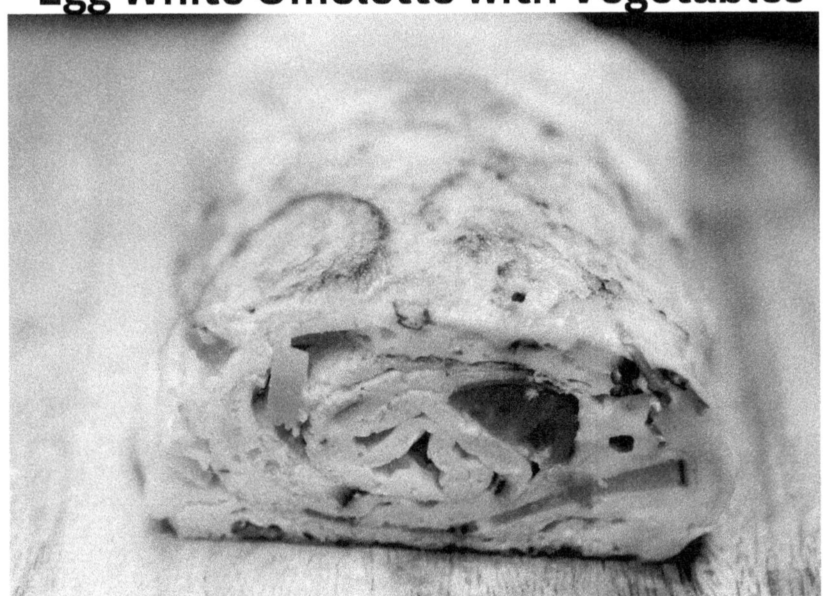

Ingredients

- 4 egg whites
- 1/2 bell pepper, diced
- 1/2 onion, diced
- Handful of spinach leaves
- Salt and pepper to taste
- Cooking spray

Instructions

1. Whisk egg whites and season with salt and pepper.
2. Spray a skillet with cooking spray and sauté vegetables until tender.
3. Pour egg whites over vegetables, cook until set, and fold.
4. Serve your vegetable-packed omelette.

Nutritional Value

Calories: 150,
Protein: 20g,
Vitamins and Minerals:
Abundant in colorful
vegetables.

Brief Description/Backstory

A protein-packed egg white omelette filled with colorful vegetables, providing a low-calorie and nutritious breakfast option.

Coconut and Almond Flour Pancakes

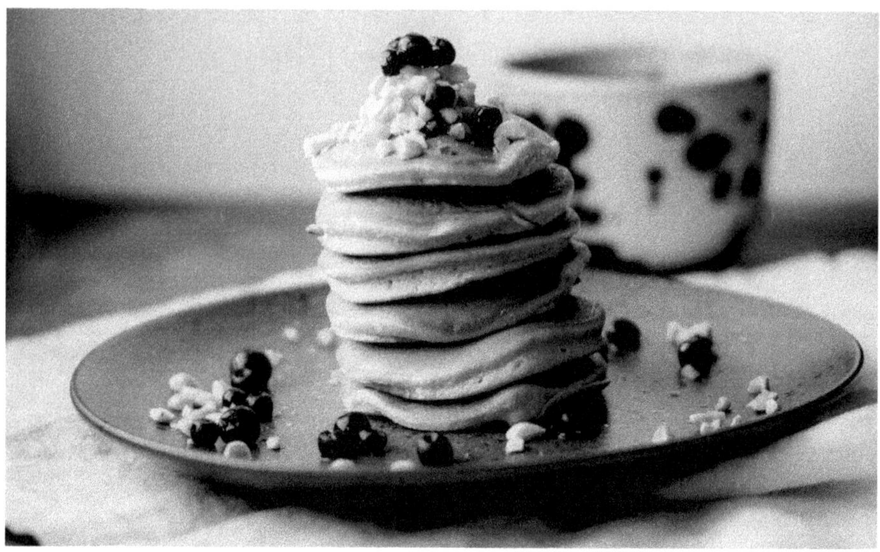

Ingredients

- 1/2 cup coconut flour
- 1/2 cup almond flour
- - 2 eggs
- 1 cup unsweetened almond milk
- 1 teaspoon baking powder
- Berries for topping

Instructions

1. Mix coconut flour, almond flour, eggs, almond milk, and baking powder.
2. Let the batter rest for 5 minutes.
3. Cook pancakes on a griddle until golden.
4. Top with berries and enjoy your guilt-free pancakes.

Nutritional Value

Calories: 250,
Protein: 10g,
Healthy Fats: Coconut and almond flour provide healthy fats.

Brief Description/Backstory

Delicious and fluffy pancakes made with coconut and almond flour, offering a gluten-free and sugarless alternative for a guilt-free breakfast treat.

Smoked Salmon and Avocado Toast

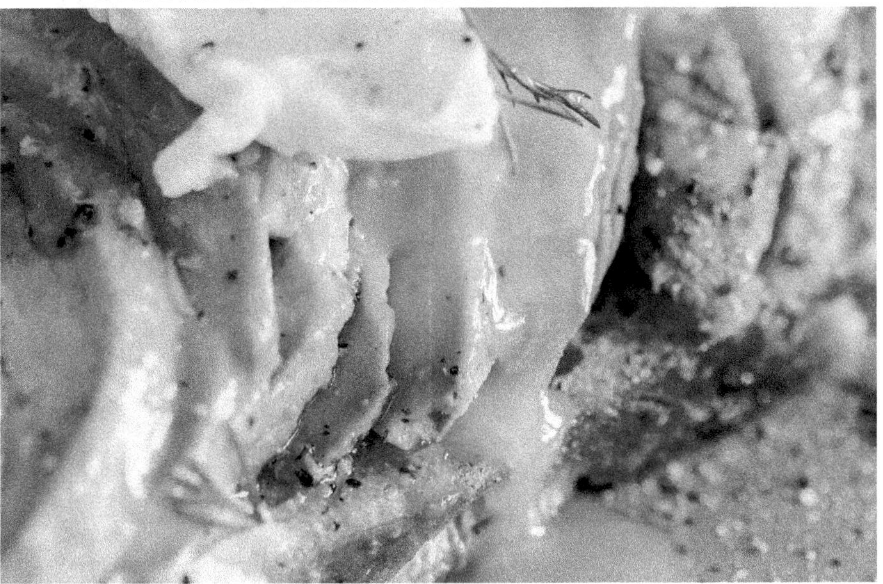

Ingredients

- 4 slices whole-grain bread, toasted
- 1 ripe avocado, mashed
- 100g smoked salmon
- Lemon wedges for garnish
- Fresh dill for garnish

Instructions

1 Toast whole-grain bread slices.
2. Spread mashed avocado on each slice.
3. Top with smoked salmon.
4. Garnish with fresh dill and a squeeze of lemon.
5. Relish your gourmet breakfast toast.

Nutritional Value

Calories: 300,
Protein: 15g,
Omega-3 Fatty Acids: High from smoked salmon.

Brief Description/Backstory

An elegant and satisfying breakfast featuring smoked salmon and creamy avocado on whole-grain toast, offering a burst of flavors and omega-3 fatty acids.

Blueberry Almond Smoothie Bowl

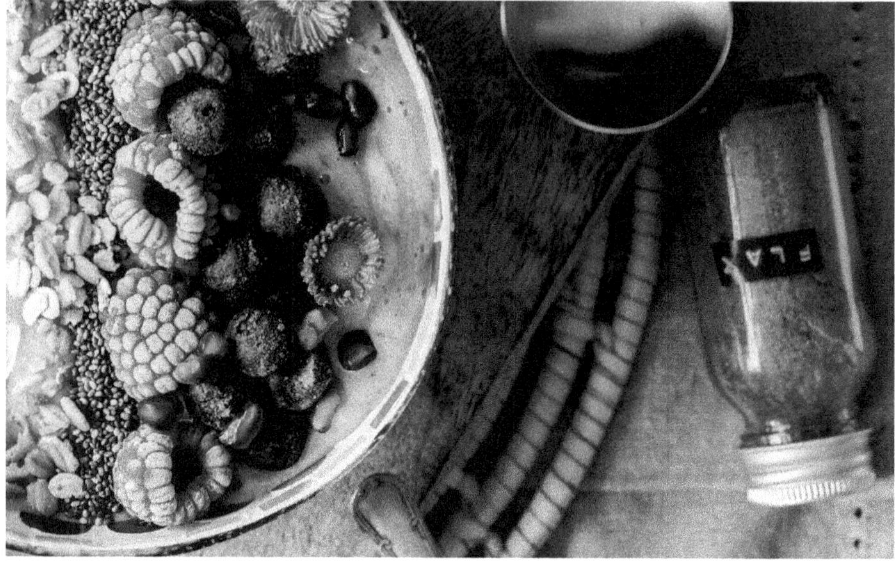

Ingredients

- 2 cups frozen blueberries
- 1 banana
- 1 cup unsweetened almond milk
- Toppings: Almonds, chia seeds, fresh blueberries

Instructions

1. Blend frozen blueberries, banana, and almond milk until smooth.
2. Pour into bowls and add desired toppings.
3. Dive into a delightful blueberry almond smoothie bowl.

Nutritional Value

Calories: 250,
Fiber: 8g,
Antioxidants: Blueberries are rich in antioxidants.

Brief Description/Backstory

A vibrant smoothie bowl featuring antioxidant-rich blueberries, almond milk, and nutritious toppings for a delicious and nutritious breakfast.

Turmeric and Spinach Scrambled Eggs

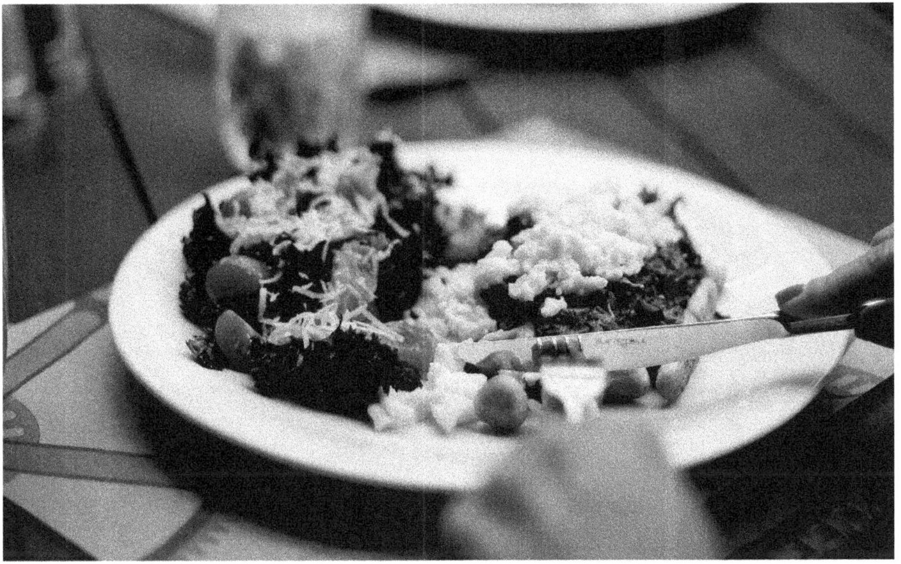

Ingredients

- 4 eggs
- 1 teaspoon ground turmeric
- Handful of fresh spinach, chopped
- Salt and pepper to taste

Instructions

1. Whisk eggs and add ground turmeric.
2. Cook eggs in a skillet until slightly set.
3. Add chopped spinach and continue cooking until eggs are fully cooked.
4. Season with salt and pepper.
5. Savor your turmeric and spinach scrambled eggs.

Nutritional Value

Calories: 200,
Protein: 18g,
Anti-Inflammatory:
Turmeric provides anti-inflammatory properties.

Brief Description/Backstory

A savory twist on traditional scrambled eggs, featuring the anti-inflammatory benefits of turmeric and the nutrient boost from fresh spinach.

Lunch Creations

These sugarless lunch creations offer a variety of flavors and textures, proving that nutritious meals can be delicious and satisfying. From colorful salads to comforting soups, these recipes are designed to elevate your lunchtime experience while supporting your health and well-being. Enjoy the wholesome goodness of these sugarless lunch options!

Quinoa Salad with Roasted Vegetables

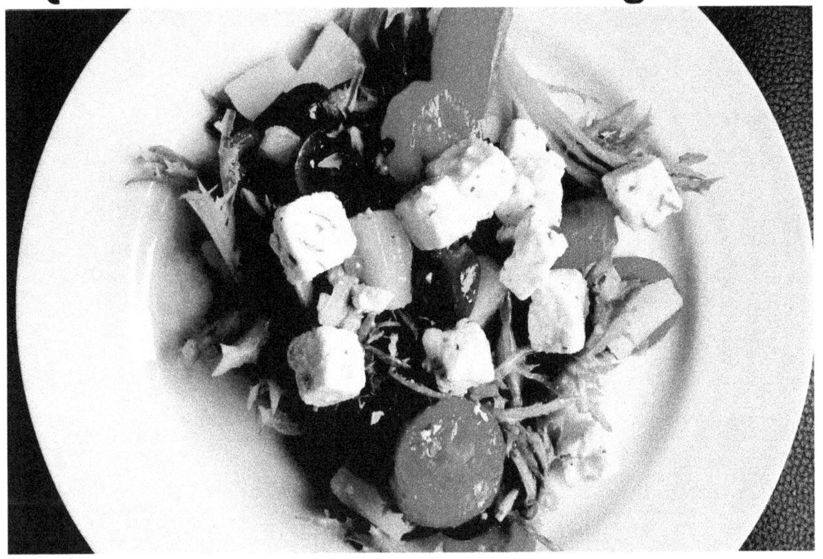

Ingredients

- cup quinoa, cooked
- Assorted vegetables (bell peppers, zucchini, cherry tomatoes)
- Olive oil for roasting
- Fresh herbs (parsley, basil)
- Balsamic vinaigrette dressing

Instructions

1. Toss vegetables in olive oil, roast until tender.
2. Mix quinoa and roasted vegetables.
3. Add fresh herbs and drizzle with balsamic vinaigrette.
4. Toss gently and serve your nutrient-packed quinoa salad.

Nutritional Value

Calories: 200, Protein: 18g, Anti-Inflammatory: Turmeric provides anti-inflammatory properties.

Brief Description/Backstory

A vibrant quinoa salad featuring a medley of roasted vegetables, providing a nutritious and satisfying sugarless lunch option.

Grilled Chicken and Avocado Wrap

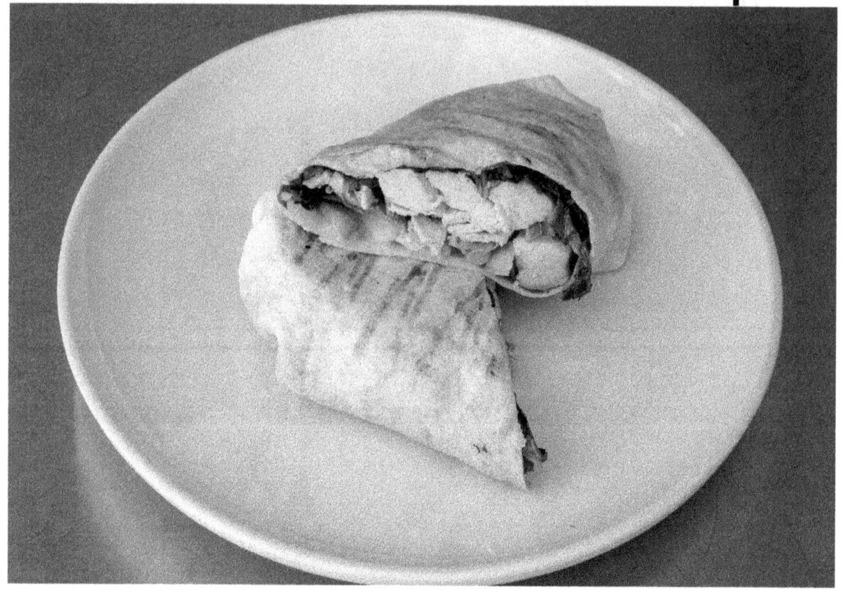

Ingredients

- 2 boneless, skinless chicken breasts
- Whole-grain wraps
- 1 ripe avocado, sliced
- Lettuce, tomato, and cucumber slices
- Greek yogurt for dressing

Instructions

1. Grill chicken breasts until fully cooked.
2. Slice chicken and assemble wraps with avocado and veggies.
3. Drizzle with Greek yogurt as a healthy dressing.
4. Roll and enjoy your grilled chicken and avocado wrap.

Nutritional Value

Calories: 400,
Protein: 25g,
Healthy Fats: Avocado provides monounsaturated fats.

Brief Description/Backstory

A protein-rich wrap featuring grilled chicken, creamy avocado, and crisp vegetables for a wholesome and sugarless lunch.

Chickpea and Vegetable Stir-Fry

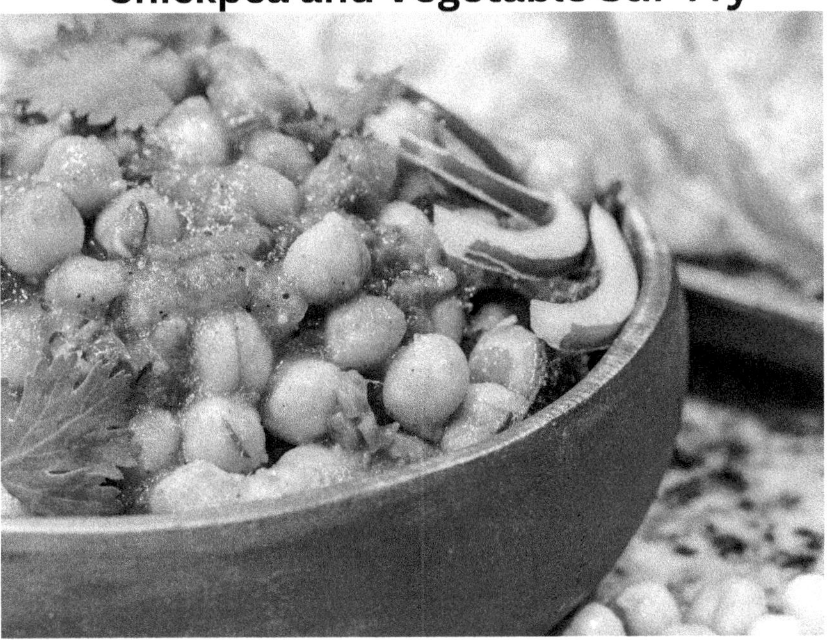

Ingredients

- 2 cans chickpeas, drained and rinsed
- Assorted vegetables (broccoli, bell peppers, snap peas)
- Soy sauce for seasoning
- Garlic and ginger for flavor
- Brown rice for serving

Instructions

1. Sauté garlic and ginger, add vegetables and chickpeas.
2. Stir-fry until vegetables are tender.
3. Season with soy sauce.
4. Serve over brown rice and enjoy your chickpea stir-fry.

Nutritional Value

Calories: 350,
Protein: 15g,
Fiber: 10g,
Iron: High.

Brief Description/Backstory

A flavorful and fiber-rich stir-fry featuring chickpeas and a colorful array of vegetables, providing a satisfying and sugarless lunch option.

Salmon and Asparagus Foil Packets

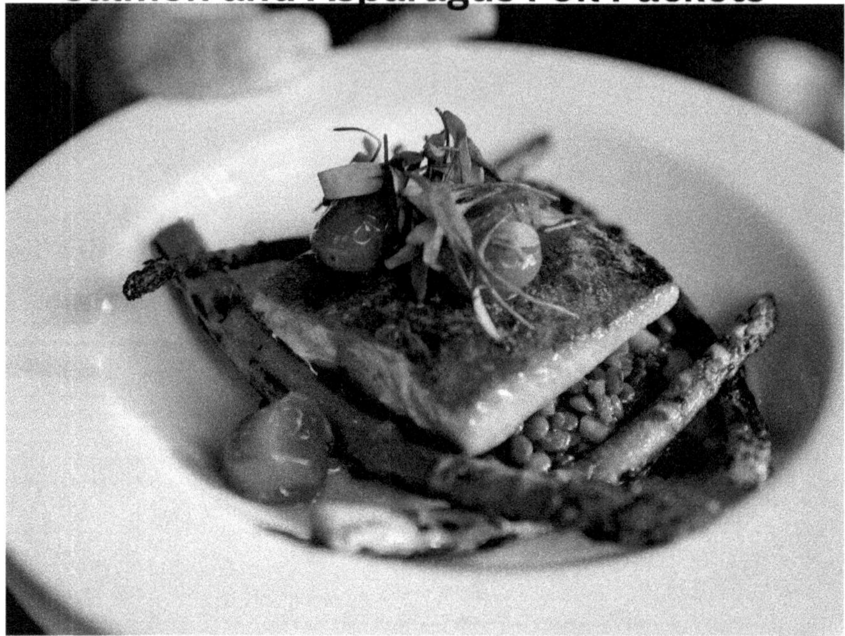

Ingredients

- 2 salmon fillets
- Fresh asparagus spears
- Lemon slices
- Olive oil for drizzling
- Fresh dill for seasoning

Instructions

1. Place salmon fillets and asparagus on foil.
2. Drizzle with olive oil, add lemon slices and fresh dill.
3. Seal foil packets and bake until salmon is cooked.
4. Unwrap and savor your salmon and asparagus foil packets.

Nutritional Value

Calories: 350,
Protein: 25g,
Omega-3 Fatty Acids: High.

Brief Description/Backstory

A simple and nutritious lunch option featuring salmon fillets and asparagus cooked to perfection in foil packets, preserving flavors without added sugars.

Mushroom and Spinach Quiche

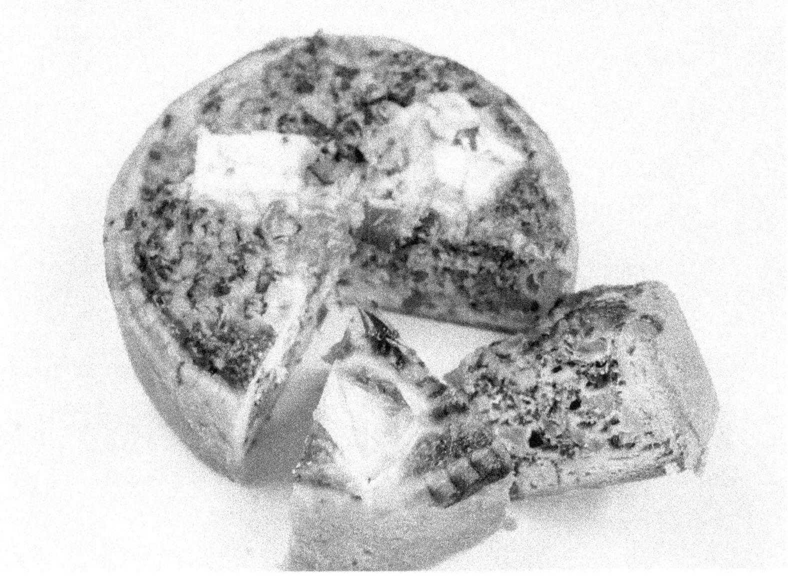

Ingredients

- 1 pie crust (store-bought or homemade)
- 1 cup mushrooms, sliced
- 2 cups fresh spinach
- - 4 eggs
- 1 cup milk (dairy or plant-based)
- Salt, pepper, and nutmeg for seasoning

Nutritional Value

Calories: 300,
Protein: 15g,
Iron: High,
Vitamins: A, C.

Instructions

1. Pre-bake pie crust according to instructions.
2. Sauté mushrooms and spinach until wilted.
3. Whisk eggs, add milk, salt, pepper, and nutmeg.
4. Mix in sautéed vegetables and pour into the pie crust.
5. Bake until the quiche is set and golden.

Brief Description/Backstory

A savory and sugarless quiche filled with earthy mushrooms and nutrient-packed spinach, offering a delightful lunch option.

Lentil and Vegetable Soup

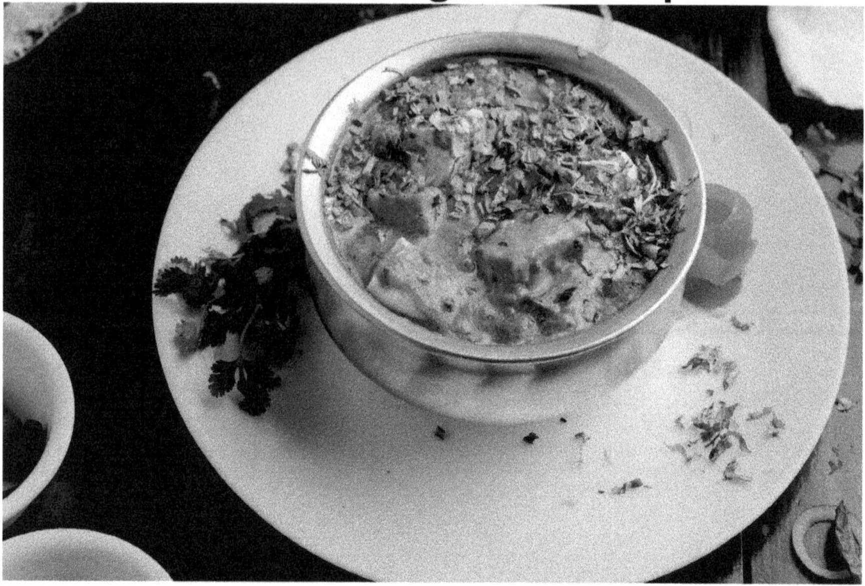

Ingredients

- 1 cup dried green lentils
- Assorted vegetables (carrots, celery, tomatoes)
- Vegetable broth
- Garlic and cumin for flavor
- Fresh parsley for garnish

Instructions

1. Rinse lentils and cook until tender.
2. Sauté garlic, add vegetables and lentils.
3. Pour in vegetable broth and simmer.
4. Season with cumin and garnish with fresh parsley.
5. Serve your hearty lentil and vegetable soup

Nutritional Value

Calories: 250,
Protein: 15g,
Fiber: 12g,
Vitamin A: High.

Brief Description/Backstory

A hearty and wholesome soup featuring lentils, vegetables, and aromatic spices for a comforting and sugarless lunch.

Eggplant and Zucchini Lasagna

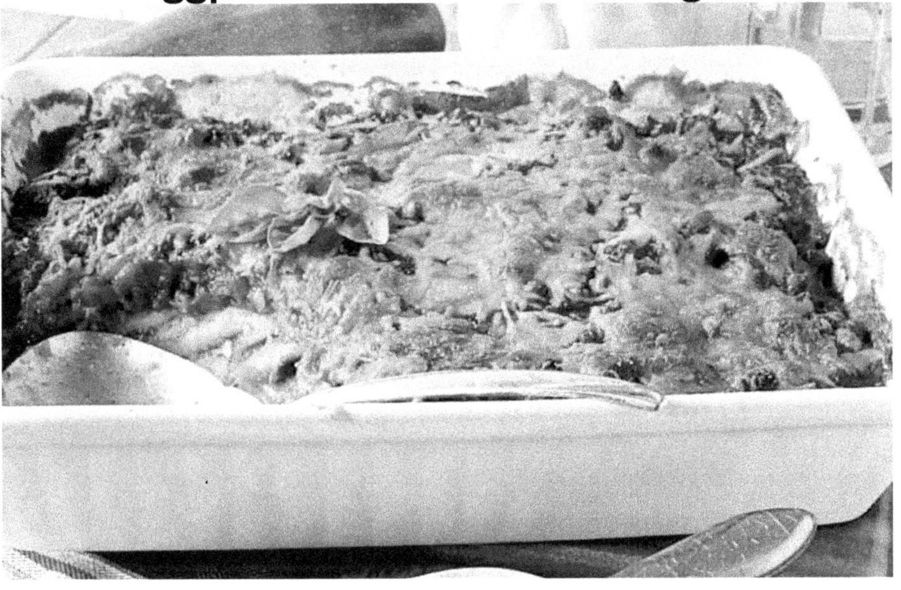

Ingredients

- 1 large eggplant, sliced
- 2 medium zucchinis, sliced
- Tomato sauce (no added sugar)
- Ricotta cheese
- Parmesan cheese for topping

Instructions

1. Roast eggplant and zucchini slices until tender.
2. Layer with tomato sauce and ricotta in a baking dish.
3. Repeat layers and top with Parmesan cheese.
4. Bake until bubbly and golden.
5. Enjoy your eggplant and zucchini lasagna.

Nutritional Value

Calories: 280,
Protein: 14g,
Fiber: 8g.

Brief Description/Backstory

A wholesome and sugarless twist on traditional lasagna, featuring layers of roasted eggplant and zucchini with a savory tomato sauce and ricotta.

Shrimp and Vegetable Skewers

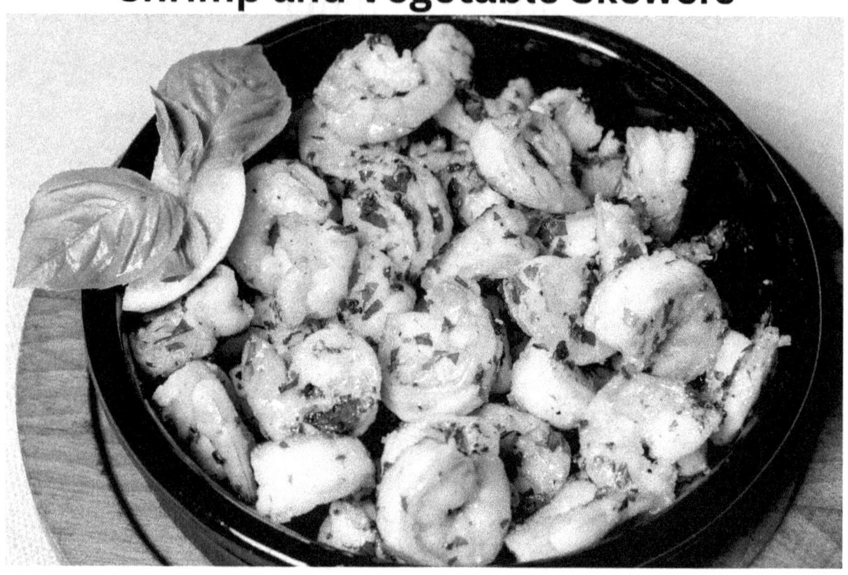

Ingredients

- 1 pound shrimp, peeled and deveined
- Assorted vegetables (bell peppers, cherry tomatoes, red onion)
- Olive oil for marinating
- Lemon wedges for garnish

Instructions

1. Marinate shrimp and vegetables in olive oil.
2. Thread onto skewers and grill until shrimp is cooked.
3. Garnish with lemon wedges.
4. Savor your grilled shrimp and vegetable skewers.

Nutritional Value

Calories: 200,
Protein: 20g,
Vitamin C: High.

Brief Description/Backstory

A flavorful and low-calorie lunch option featuring grilled shrimp and a colorful assortment of vegetables, providing a satisfying and sugarless meal.

Cauliflower and Chickpea Curry

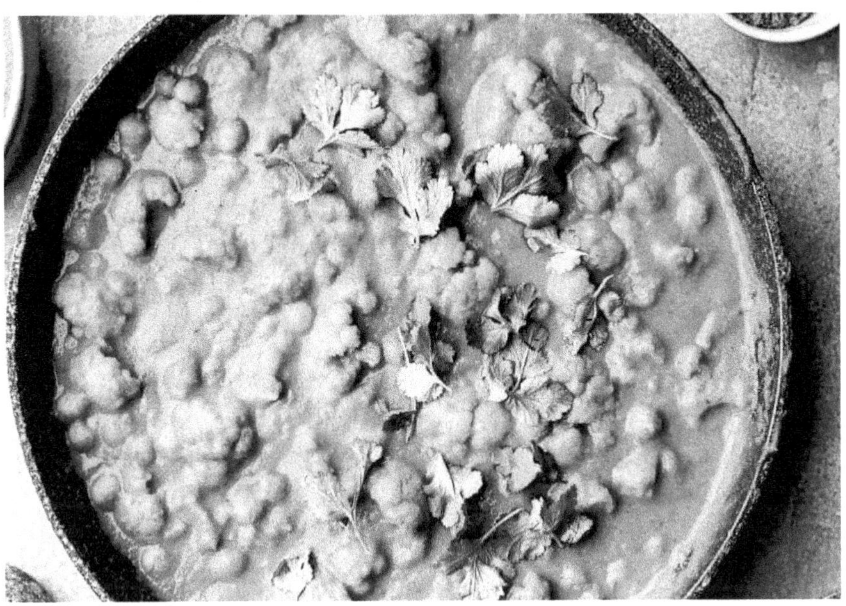

Ingredients

- 1 cauliflower, cut into florets
- 2 cans chickpeas, drained
- Curry spices (turmeric, cumin, coriander)
- Coconut milk for creaminess
- Fresh cilantro for garnish

Instructions

1. Sauté cauliflower and chickpeas in curry spices.
2. Pour in coconut milk and simmer until cauliflower is tender.
3. Garnish with fresh cilantro.
4. Serve your cauliflower and chickpea curry over rice.

Nutritional Value

Calories: 300,
Protein: 12g,
Fiber: 10g.

Brief Description/Backstory

A flavorful and sugarless curry featuring cauliflower and chickpeas, enriched with aromatic spices for a hearty and satisfying lunch.

Caprese Stuffed Portobello Mushrooms

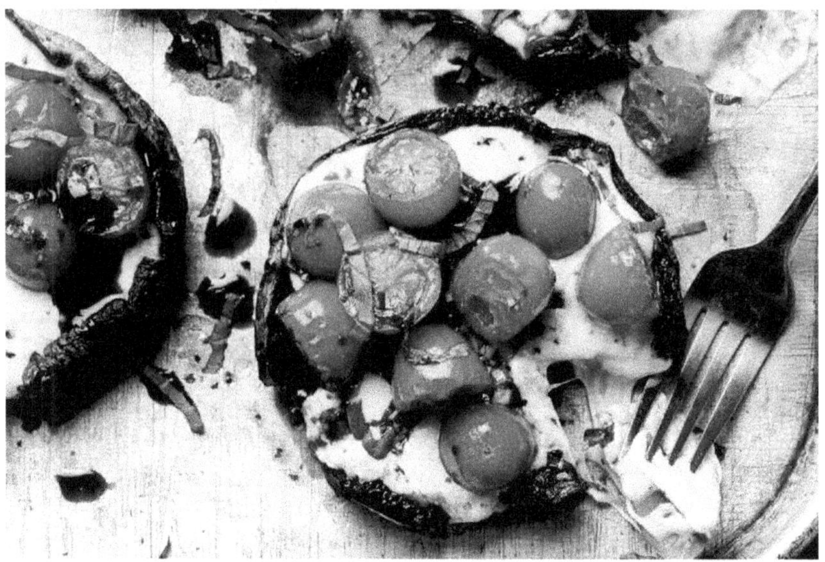

Ingredients

- 4 large portobello mushrooms
- Fresh tomatoes, sliced
- Fresh mozzarella, sliced
- Fresh basil leaves
- Balsamic glaze for drizzling

Instructions

1. Clean portobello mushrooms and remove stems.
2. Layer with sliced tomatoes, mozzarella, and basil.
3. Drizzle with balsamic glaze.
4. Bake until mushrooms are tender.
5. Savor your Caprese stuffed portobello mushrooms.

Nutritional Value

Calories: 220,
Protein: 15g,
Healthy Fats: Mozzarella provides healthy fats.

Brief Description/Backstory

A delightful and sugarless twist on the classic Caprese salad, featuring portobello mushrooms stuffed with fresh tomatoes, mozzarella, and basil.

Dinner Sensations

These sugarless dinner sensations showcase a diverse range of flavors and ingredients, proving that wholesome meals can be both delicious and satisfying. From grilled kebabs to comforting casseroles, these recipes offer a variety of options to make your dinner a delightful and nutritious experience. Enjoy these flavorful and sugar-free dinner creations!

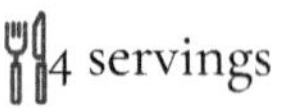

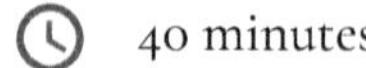

Baked Lemon Herb Chicken

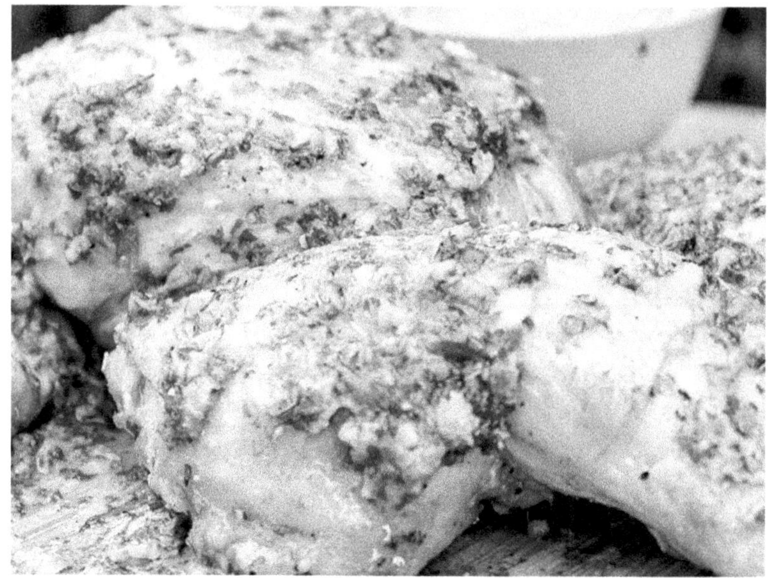

Ingredients

- 4 boneless, skinless chicken breasts
- Fresh herbs (rosemary, thyme, parsley)
- Zest and juice of 1 lemon
- Olive oil
- Salt and pepper to taste

Instructions

1. Preheat oven to 375°F (190°C).
2. Season chicken breasts with salt, pepper, and herbs.
3. Drizzle with olive oil and lemon juice.
4. Bake until chicken is cooked through and golden.
5. Garnish with lemon zest and fresh herbs.

Nutritional Value

Calories: 250,
Protein: 30g,
Vitamin C: High.

Brief Description/Backstory

A zesty and succulent baked chicken dish infused with fresh herbs and citrusy flavors, making it a delightful and sugarless dinner sensation.

Spaghetti Squash Primavera

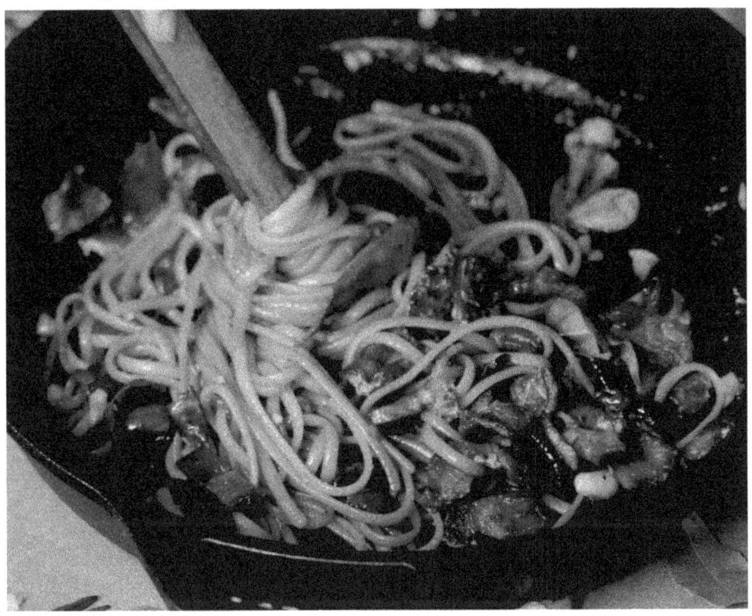

Ingredients

- 1 large spaghetti squash
- Assorted vegetables (bell peppers, cherry tomatoes, broccoli)
- Olive oil for roasting
- Marinara sauce (no added sugar)
- Fresh basil for garnish

Instructions

1. Cut spaghetti squash in half, remove seeds, and roast until tender.
2. Roast vegetables in olive oil until lightly caramelized.
3. Scrape spaghetti squash strands and toss with roasted vegetables.
4. Warm marinara sauce and pour over the squash mixture.
5. Garnish with fresh basil and serve.

Nutritional Value

Calories: 180,
Fiber: 8g,
Vitamins: A, C.

Brief Description/Backstory

A low-carb alternative to traditional pasta, this spaghetti squash primavera is a vegetable-packed dinner sensation with a medley of vibrant flavors.

Grilled Mahi-Mahi with Mango Salsa

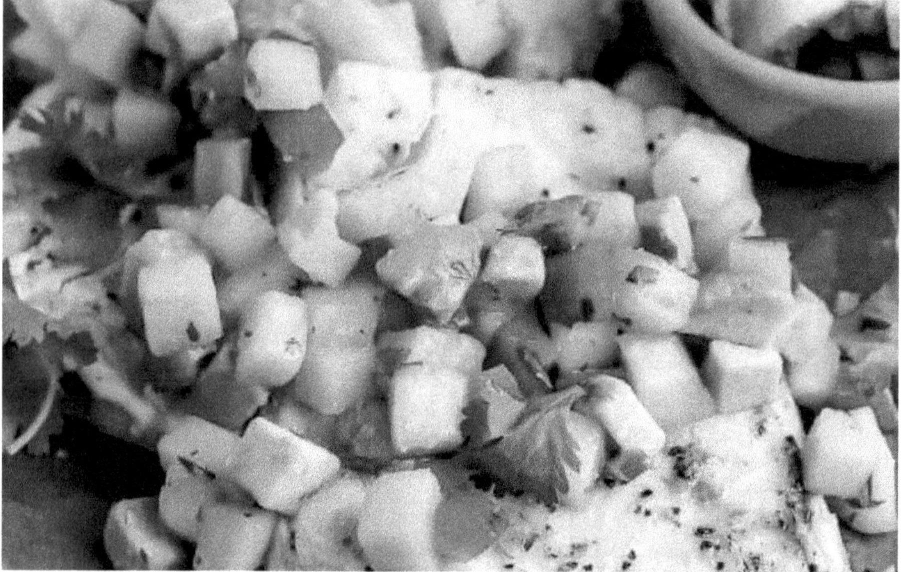

Ingredients

- 4 mahi-mahi fillets
- 2 ripe mangoes, diced
- Red onion, finely chopped
- Fresh cilantro
- Lime juice
- Salt and pepper to taste

Instructions

1. Season mahi-mahi with salt and pepper and grill until cooked.
2. Mix diced mango, red onion, cilantro, and lime juice for salsa.
3. Top grilled fish with mango salsa.
4. Serve your grilled mahi-mahi with a burst of tropical flavors.

Nutritional Value

Calories: 220,
Protein: 25g,
Vitamin C: High.

Brief Description/Backstory

A tropical delight featuring grilled mahi-mahi topped with vibrant mango salsa, creating a flavorful and sugarless dinner sensation.

Cauliflower Fried Rice with Shrimp

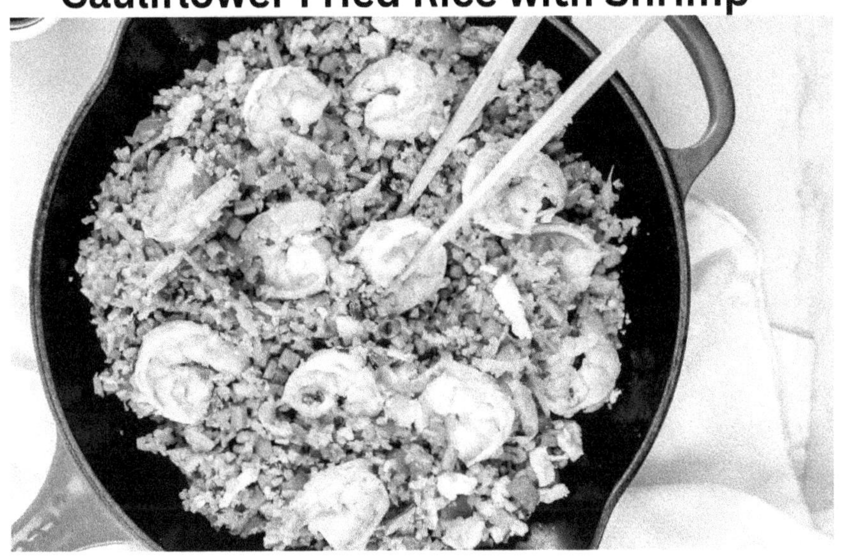

Ingredients

- 1 medium cauliflower, grated
- 1 pound shrimp, peeled and deveined
- Mixed vegetables (peas, carrots, corn)
- Soy sauce for seasoning
- Scallions for garnish

Nutritional Value

Calories: 180,
Protein: 20g,
Fiber: 5g.

Instructions

1. Sauté grated cauliflower in a pan until tender.
2. Add shrimp and mixed vegetables, cook until shrimp is pink.
3. Season with soy sauce.
4. Garnish with scallions and serve.

Brief Description/Backstory

A low-carb twist on classic fried rice, this cauliflower fried rice with shrimp is a delicious and sugarless dinner option with plenty of savory flavors.

Stuffed Bell Peppers with Turkey and Quinoa

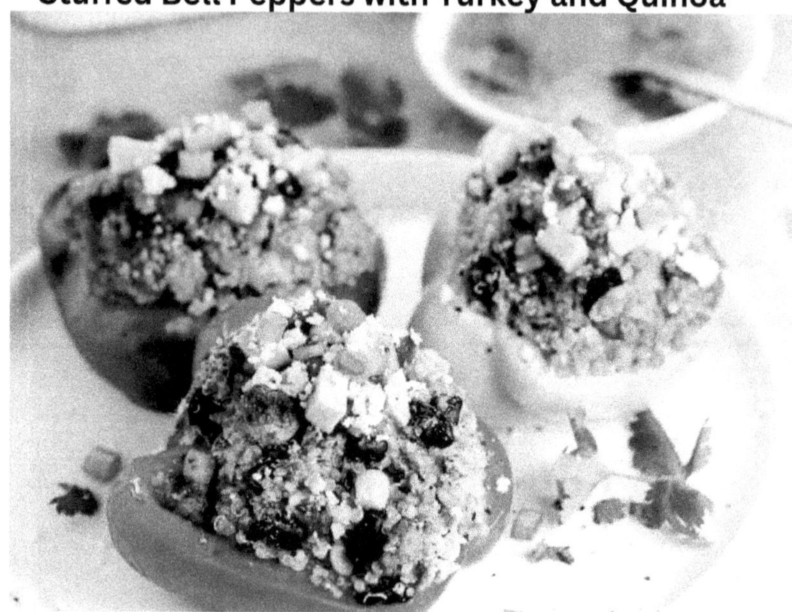

Ingredients

- 4 bell peppers, halved
- 1 pound ground turkey
- 1 cup cooked quinoa
- Tomato sauce (no added sugar)
- Italian herbs for seasoning
- Mozzarella cheese for topping

Instructions

1. Preheat oven to 375°F (190°C).
2. Brown ground turkey, mix with cooked quinoa and tomato sauce.
3. Season with Italian herbs.
4. Stuff bell pepper halves with the turkey and quinoa mixture.
5. Top with mozzarella cheese and bake until bubbly.

Nutritional Value

Calories: 300,
Protein: 25g,
Fiber: 7g.

Brief Description/Backstory

A wholesome and protein-packed dinner option, these stuffed bell peppers with turkey and quinoa are a balanced and sugarless delight.

Salmon and Vegetable Kebabs

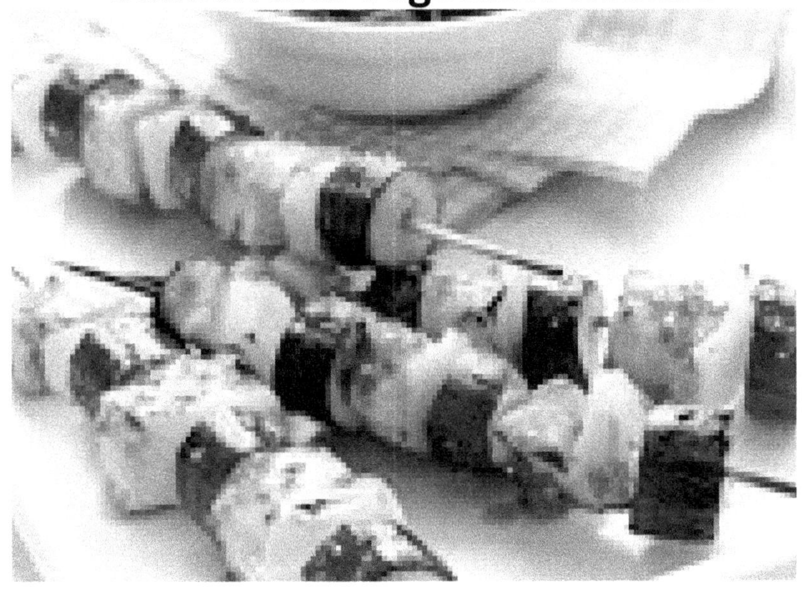

Ingredients

- 1 pound salmon fillets, cut into cubes
- Assorted vegetables (bell peppers, cherry tomatoes, red onion)
- Olive oil for marinating
- Lemon wedg

Instructions

1. Marinate salmon cubes and vegetables in olive oil.
2. Thread onto skewers and grill until salmon is cooked.
3. Garnish with lemon wedges.
4. Enjoy your grilled salmon and vegetable kebabs.

Nutritional Value

Calories: 250,
Protein: 22g,
Omega-3 Fatty Acids: High.

Brief Description/Backstory

A delightful and colorful dinner sensation, these salmon and vegetable kebabs are grilled to perfection, offering a healthy and sugarless option for seafood lovers.

Vegetarian Eggplant Lasagna

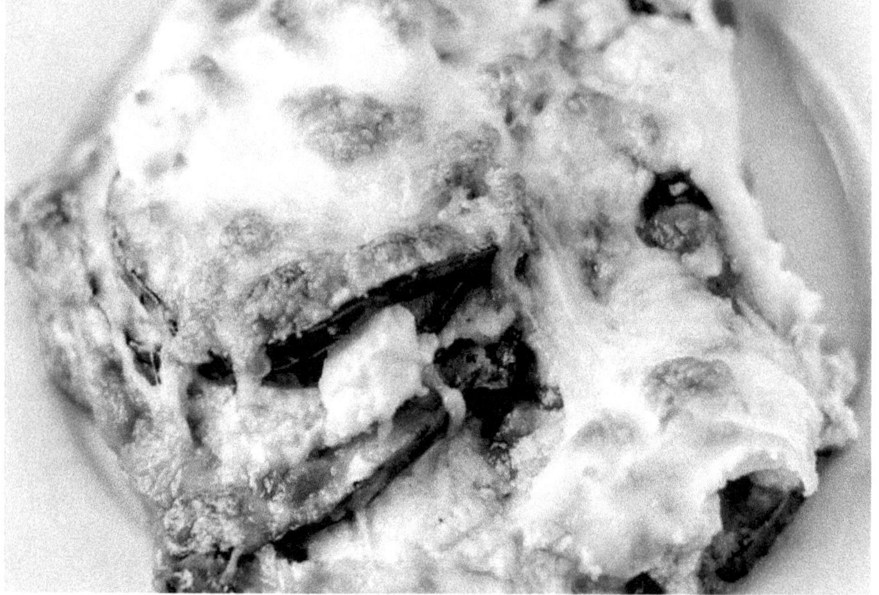

Ingredients

- 2 large eggplants, sliced
- Tomato sauce (no added sugar)
- Ricotta cheese
- Parmesan cheese for topping
- Fresh basil for garnis

Instructions

1. Roast eggplant slices until tender.
2. Layer with tomato sauce and ricotta in a baking dish.
3. Repeat layers and top with Parmesan cheese.
4. Bake until bubbly and golden.
5. Garnish with fresh basil.

Nutritional Value

Calories: 280,
Protein: 15g,
Fiber: 8g.

Brief Description/Backstory

A hearty and satisfying vegetarian dinner sensation, this eggplant lasagna is layered with roasted eggplant, rich tomato sauce, and creamy ricotta.

Mushroom and Spinach Stuffed Chicken Breast

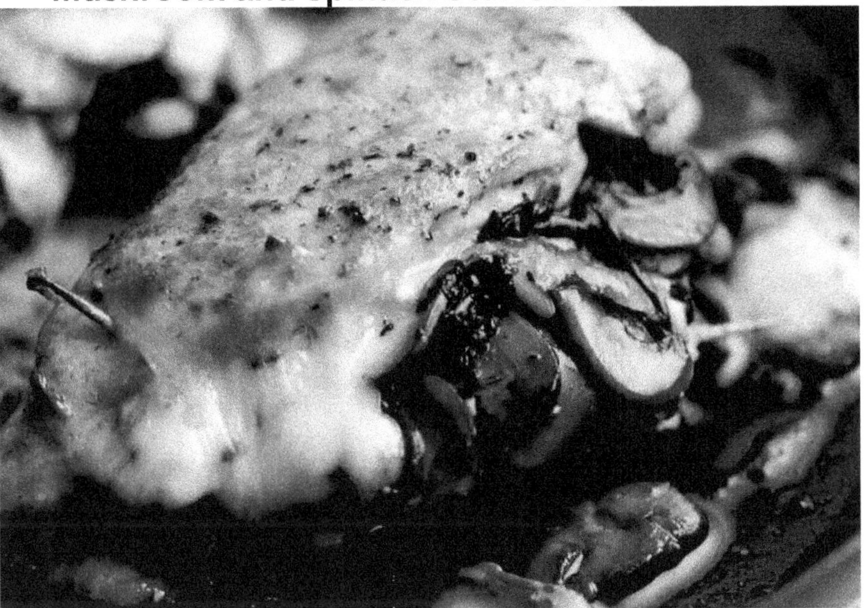

Ingredients

- 4 boneless, skinless chicken breasts
- Mushroom and spinach stuffing
- Olive oil for searing
- Chicken broth for deglazing
- Fresh thyme for garnish

Instructions

1. Butterfly chicken breasts and stuff with mushroom and spinach mixture.
2. Sear stuffed chicken in olive oil until golden.
3. Deglaze with chicken broth and bake until cooked.
4. Garnish with fresh thyme and serve.

Nutritional Value

Calories: 260,
Protein: 30g,
Iron: High.

Brief Description/Backstory

An elegant and flavorful dinner option, these mushroom and spinach stuffed chicken breasts are a delectable and sugarless way to elevate your meal.

Cabbage and Turkey Stir-Fry

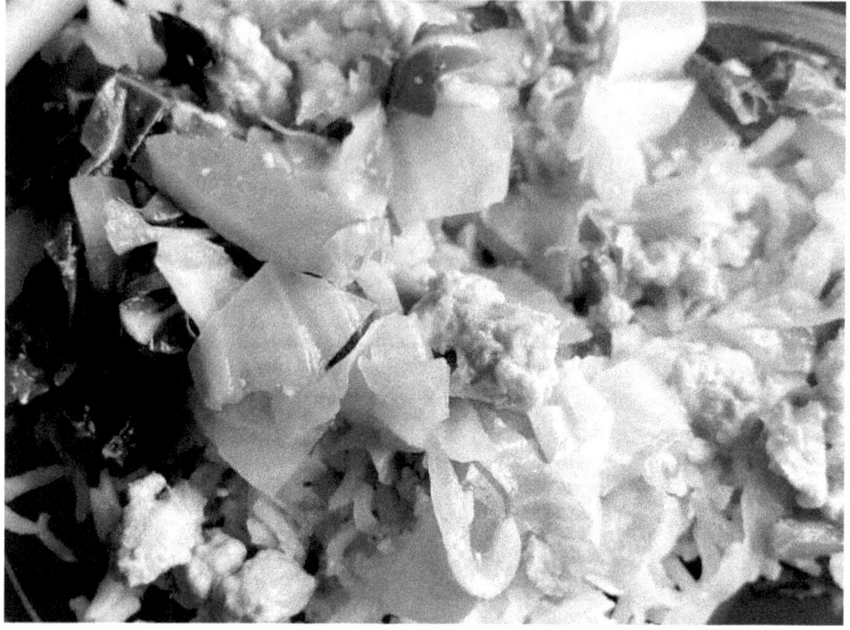

Ingredients

- 1 small cabbage, shredded
- 1 pound ground turkey
- Soy sauce for seasoning
- Ginger and garlic for flavor
- Green onions for garnish

Instructions

1. Sauté ground turkey until browned.
2. Add shredded cabbage and stir-fry until tender-crisp.
3. Season with soy sauce, ginger, and garlic.
4. Garnish with green onions and serve.

Nutritional Value

Calories: 220,
Protein: 25g,
Fiber: 6g.

Brief Description/Backstory

A quick and flavorful dinner sensation, this cabbage and turkey stir-fry is a low-carb and sugarless option with a perfect blend of savory and crunchy textures.

Zucchini Noodles with Pesto and Cherry Tomatoes

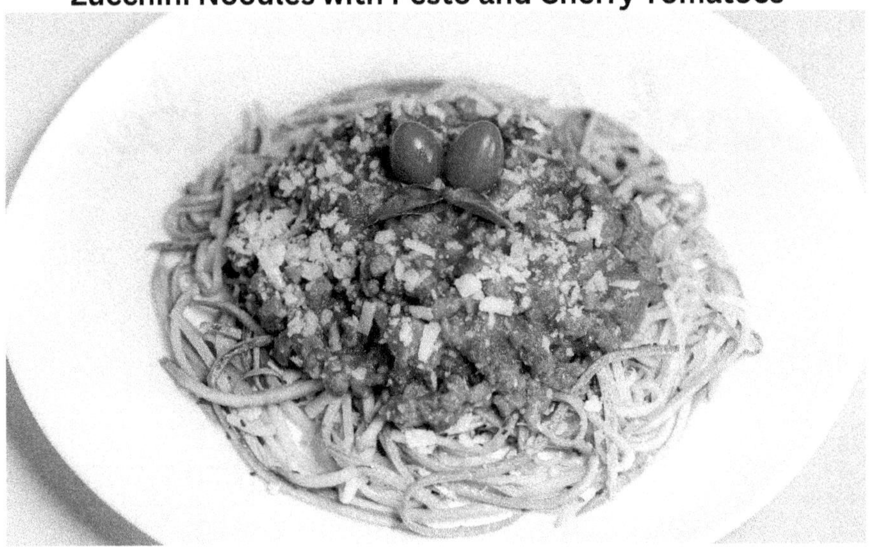

Ingredients

- 4 zucchinis, spiralized
- Pesto sauce (homemade or store-bought)
- Cherry tomatoes, halved
- Pine nuts for garnish
- Fresh basil for garnish

Instructions

1. Spiralize zucchinis into noodle-like strands.
2. Toss zucchini noodles with pesto sauce.
3. Top with cherry tomatoes, pine nuts, and fresh basil.
4. Enjoy your light and vibrant zucchini noodle dish.

Nutritional Value

Calories: 180,
Fiber: 5g,
Healthy Fats: Pesto provides healthy fats.

Brief Description/Backstory

A light and refreshing dinner sensation, these zucchini noodles with pesto and cherry tomatoes offer a flavorful and sugarless alternative to traditional pasta.

snack time favorites

These sugarless snack time favorites offer a range of textures and flavors to keep your cravings satisfied in a healthy way. Whether you prefer savory or sweet, these recipes provide delicious alternatives without compromising on taste. Enjoy these guilt-free and nutritious snacks to keep you energized throughout the day!

Almond and Chia Seed Energy Bites

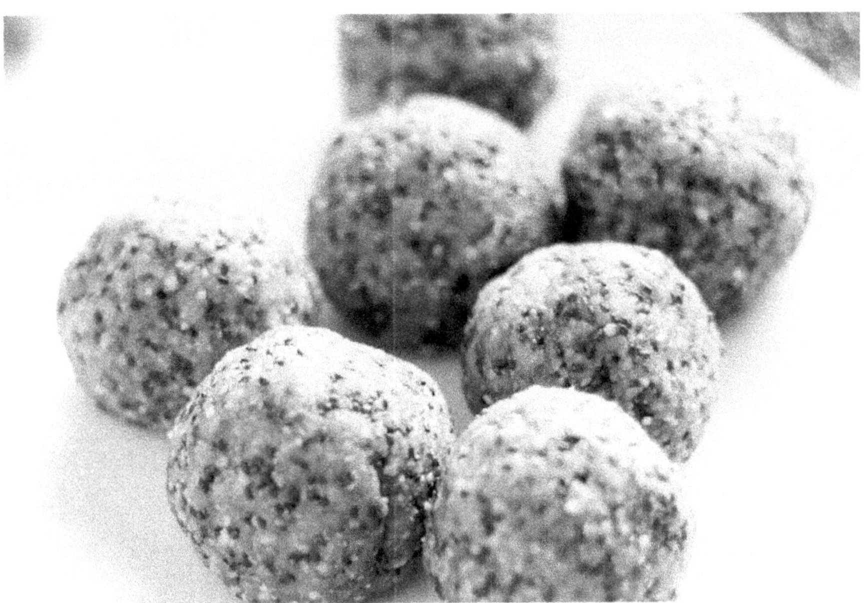

Ingredients

- 1 cup almonds
- 1/2 cup chia seeds
- 1/3 cup nut butter (almond or peanut)
- 1/4 cup honey or maple syrup
- 1 teaspoon vanilla extract

Instructions

1. In a food processor, blend almonds until finely chopped.
2. Add chia seeds, nut butter, honey or maple syrup, and vanilla extract. Pulse until well combined.
3. Roll mixture into bite-sized balls.
4. Refrigerate for at least 30 minutes before serving.

Nutritional Value

Calories: 100,
Protein: 4g,
Fiber: 3g.

Brief Description/Backstory

These almond and chia seed energy bites are a perfect snack to boost your energy and satisfy your sweet cravings without added sugars.

🍴 2 serving **Greek Yogurt and Berry Parfait**

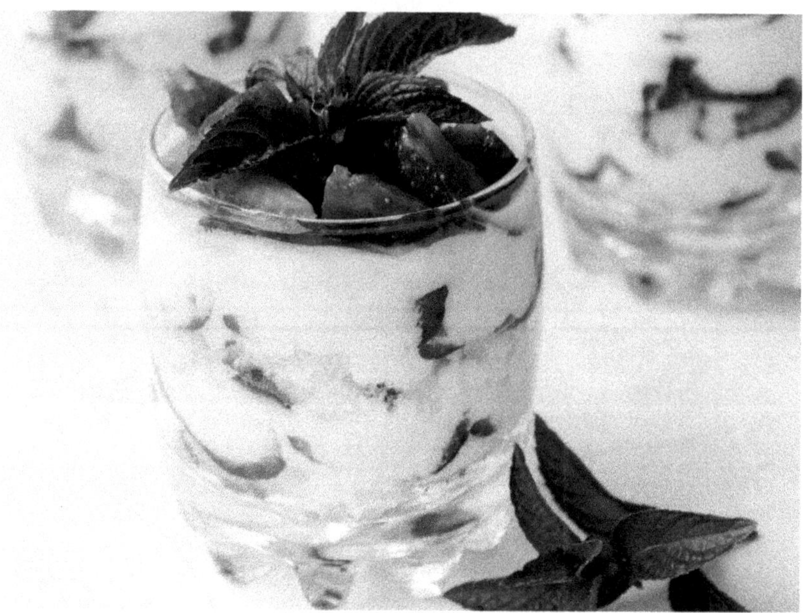

Ingredients

- 2 cups Greek yogurt
- 1 cup mixed berries (strawberries, blueberries, raspberries)
- Drizzle of honey (optional)
- Granola for crunch (sugar-free)

Instructions

1. In glasses or bowls, layer Greek yogurt and mixed berries.
2. Drizzle with honey if desired.
3. Top with sugar-free granola for added crunch.
4. Enjoy your quick and nutritious parfait.

Nutritional Value

Calories: 180,
Protein: 15g,
Probiotics:
Greek yogurt promotes gut health.

Brief Description/Backstory

A refreshing and protein-packed parfait featuring Greek yogurt and fresh berries, creating a delightful sugarless snack.

Cucumber and Hummus Bites

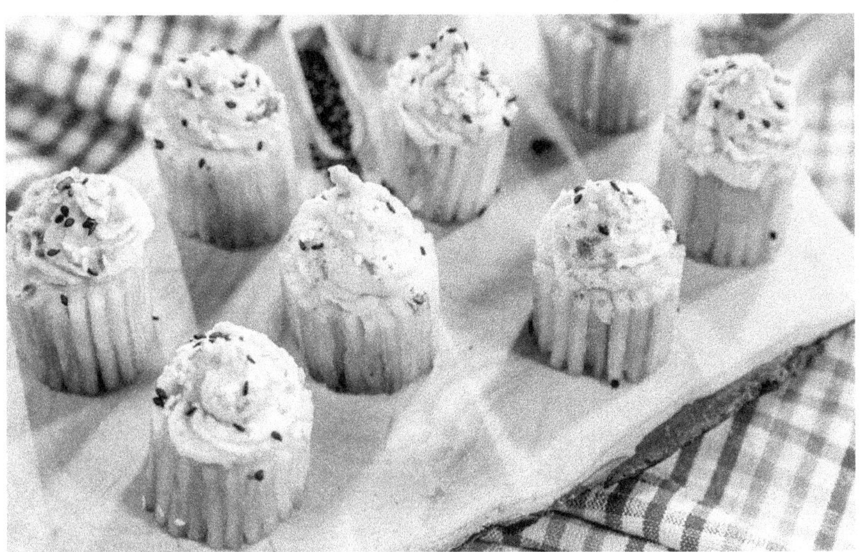

Ingredients

- 2 cucumbers, sliced
- Hummus (store-bought or homemade)
- Cherry tomatoes for garnish
- Fresh parsley for garnish

Instructions

1. Slice cucumbers into rounds.
2. Top each cucumber slice with a dollop of hummus.
3. Garnish with halved cherry tomatoes and fresh parsley.
4. Serve your refreshing cucumber and hummus bites.

Nutritional Value

Calories: 50,
Fiber: 2g.

Brief Description/Backstory

A light and hydrating snack, these cucumber and hummus bites are a perfect combination of crispness and creaminess without added sugars.

Avocado and Tomato Salsa

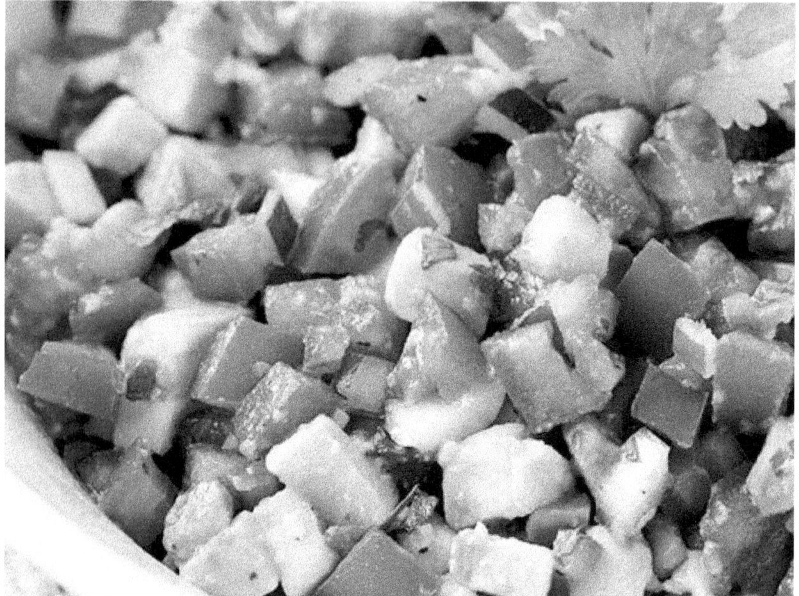

Ingredients

- 2 avocados, diced
- 1 cup cherry tomatoes, diced
- Red onion, finely chopped
- Fresh cilantro, chopped
- Lime juice
- Salt and pepper to taste

Instructions

1. In a bowl, combine diced avocados, cherry tomatoes, red onion, and cilantro.
2. Drizzle with lime juice and season with salt and pepper.
3. Mix gently and refrigerate for 10 minutes before serving.
4. Serve with vegetable sticks or whole-grain crackers.

Nutritional Value

Calories: 120, Healthy Fats: Avocado provides monounsaturated fats.

Brief Description/Backstory

A vibrant and nutrient-packed avocado and tomato salsa that serves as a delicious dip for your favorite veggies or whole-grain crackers.

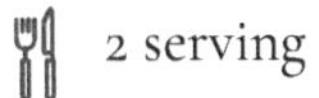 2 serving

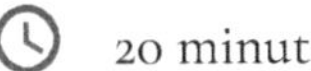 20 minutes

Kale Chips with Parmesan

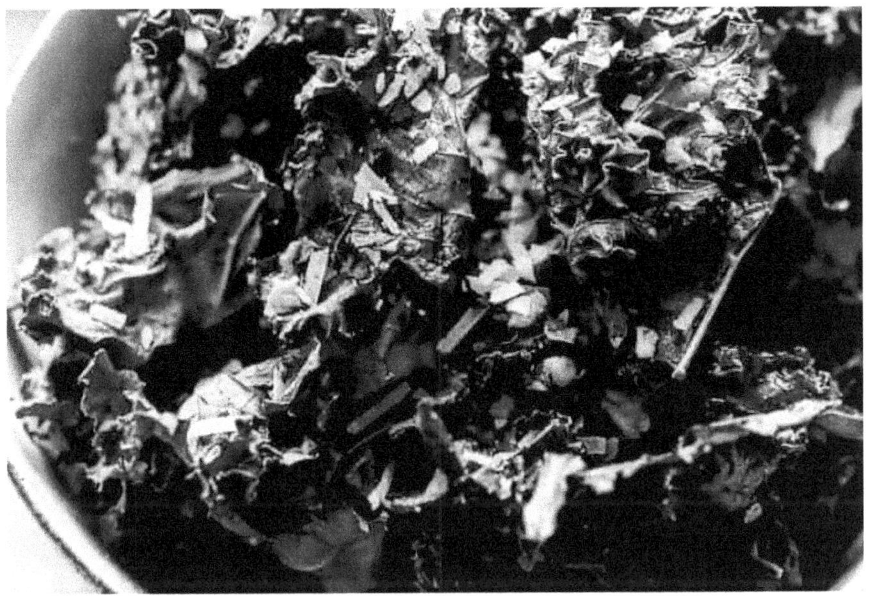

Ingredients

- 1 bunch kale, stems removed and leaves torn
- Olive oil for drizzling
- Grated Parmesan cheese
- Sea salt for seasoning

Instructions

1. Preheat oven to 350°F (175°C).
2. Massage kale leaves with olive oil.
3. Arrange on a baking sheet, sprinkle with Parmesan and sea salt.
4. Bake until crisp, about 15 minutes.
5. Enjoy your guilt-free kale chips.

Nutritional Value

Calories: 80,
Fiber: 5g,
Calcium: High.

Brief Description/Backstory

A crispy and savory snack, these kale chips with Parmesan offer a delicious way to enjoy the health benefits of kale without added sugars.

Protein-Packed Cottage Cheese and Pineapple Bowl

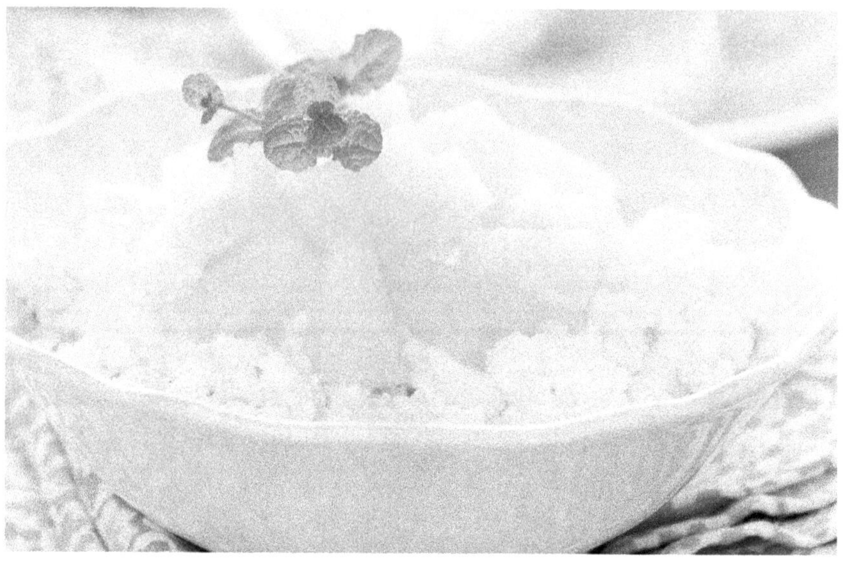

Ingredients

- 1 cup cottage cheese
- 1 cup fresh pineapple chunks
- Chopped mint for garnish
- Drizzle of honey (optional)

Instructions

1. In bowls, spoon cottage cheese and top with pineapple chunks.
2. Garnish with chopped mint and drizzle with honey if desired.
3. Enjoy the balance of creaminess and tropical sweetness.

Nutritional Value

Calories: 180,
Protein: 20g.

Brief Description/Backstory

A simple yet satisfying snack, this cottage cheese and pineapple bowl combines protein and sweetness for a delightful treat.

Turmeric Roasted Chickpeas

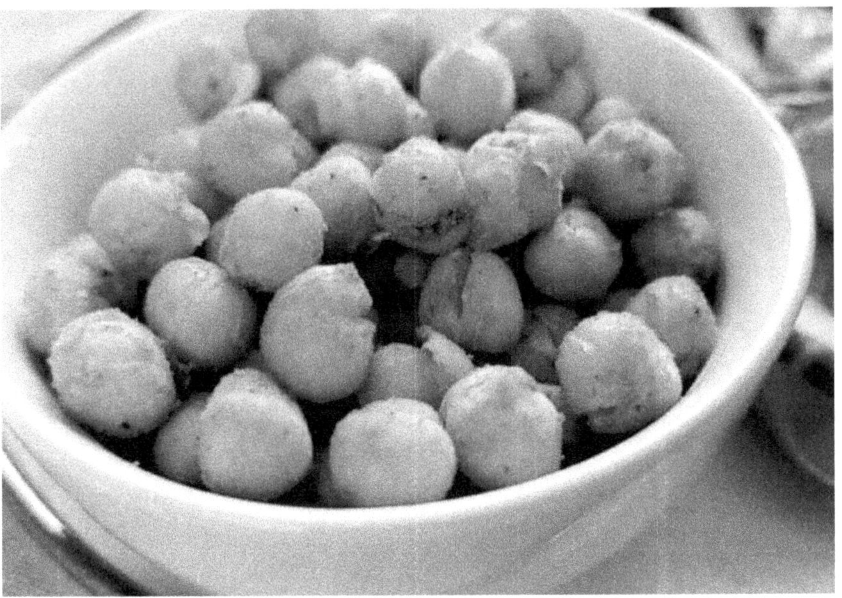

Ingredients

- 2 cans chickpeas, drained and rinsed
- Olive oil for coating
- Turmeric, cumin, and paprika for seasoning
- Salt to taste

Instructions

1. Preheat oven to 400°F (200°C).
2. Toss chickpeas with olive oil and spread on a baking sheet.
3. Season with turmeric, cumin, paprika, and salt.
4. Bake until crispy, about 30 minutes.
5. Cool before serving your turmeric roasted chickpeas.

Nutritional Value

Calories: 120,
Fiber: 6g,
Plant-Based Protein: High.

Brief Description/Backstory

A crunchy and flavorful snack, these turmeric roasted chickpeas are a wholesome alternative to processed snacks without added sugars.

Edamame and Sea Salt

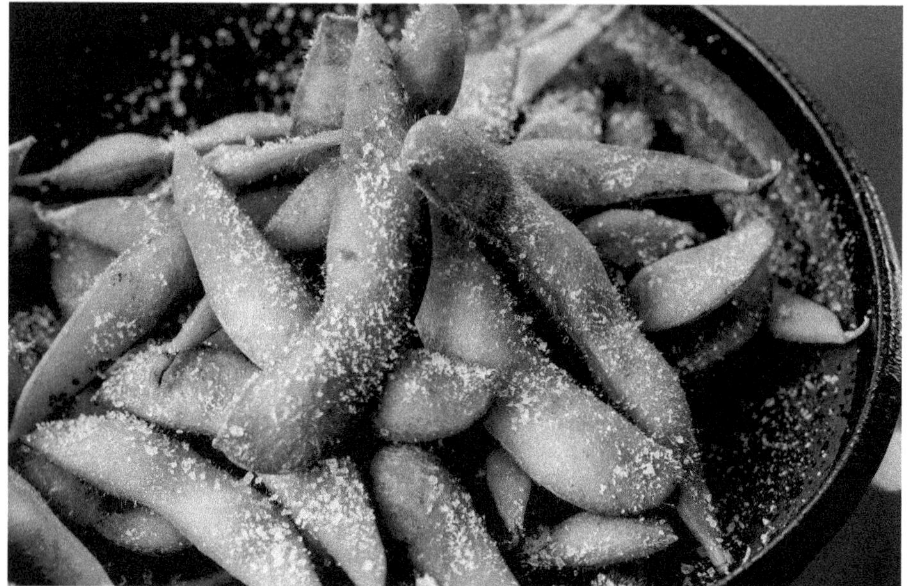

Ingredients

2 cups edamame (fresh
or frozen)
Coarse sea salt for
seasoning

Instructions

1. Boil or steam edamame
until tender.
2. Sprinkle with coarse sea
salt.
3. Toss to coat and serve.
4. Enjoy your wholesome
edamame snack.

Nutritional Value

Calories: 120,
Protein: 12g,
Fiber: 8g.

Brief Description/Backstory

A protein-packed and
satisfying snack, edamame
with sea salt is a simple yet
delicious option for those
moments when you crave a
savory bite.

Chocolate Avocado Mousse

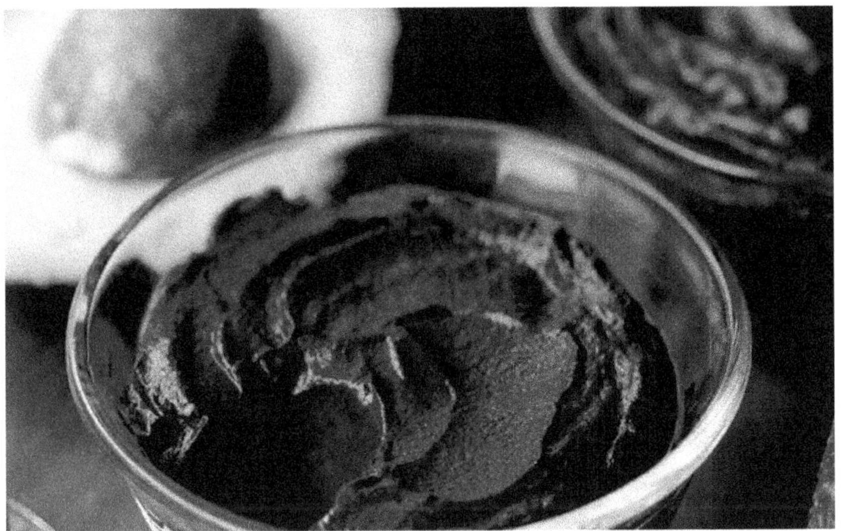

Ingredients

- 2 ripe avocados
- 1/4 cup unsweetened cocoa powder
- 1/4 cup maple syrup or honey
- 1 teaspoon vanilla extract

Instructions

1. Blend avocados, cocoa powder, maple syrup, and vanilla extract until smooth.
2. Refrigerate for at least 1 hour.
3. Spoon into bowls and enjoy your guilt-free chocolate mousse.

Nutritional Value

Calories: 150, Healthy Fats: Avocado provides monounsaturated fats.

Brief Description/Backstory

A decadent and sugarless treat, this chocolate avocado mousse combines the richness of avocado with the indulgence of dark chocolate.

🍴 4 serving

Tomato Basil Bruschetta

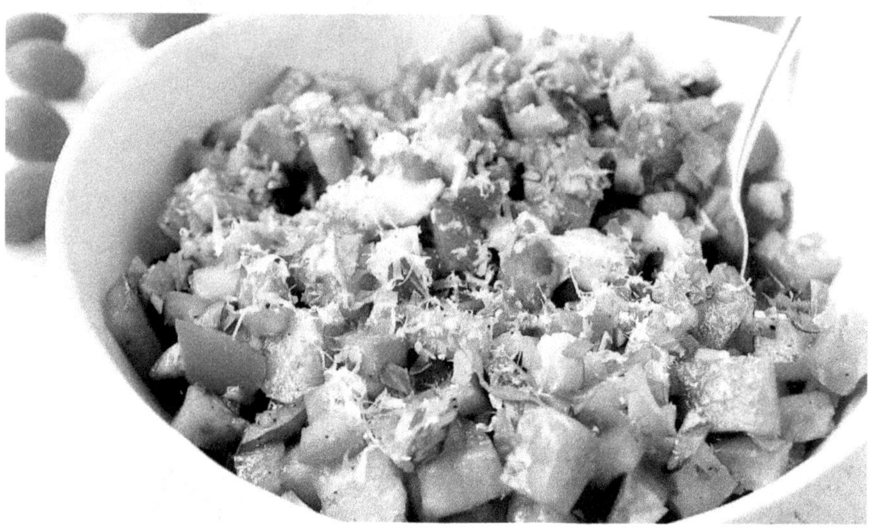

Ingredients

- 4 tomatoes, diced
- Fresh basil, chopped
- Garlic cloves, minced
- Balsamic vinegar for drizzling
- Whole-grain baguette slices

Instructions

1. In a bowl, combine diced tomatoes, fresh basil, and minced garlic.
2. Drizzle with balsamic vinegar and toss gently.
3. Toast baguette slices and top with the tomato basil mixture.
4. Serve your delightful tomato basil bruschetta.

Nutritional Value

Calories: 100,
Fiber: 3g,
Antioxidants:
Tomatoes and basil are rich in antioxidants.

Brief Description/Backstory

A classic and flavorful snack, this tomato basil bruschetta is a simple yet elegant option for those who appreciate the combination of fresh ingredients.

Dessert Indulgences

These sugarless dessert indulgences prove that you can satisfy your sweet cravings without compromising on taste or nutrition. From creamy puddings to fruity bites, these recipes offer a variety of delightful options for guilt-free dessert enjoyment. Treat yourself to these wholesome and delicious sugarless desserts!

Chocolate Avocado Pudding

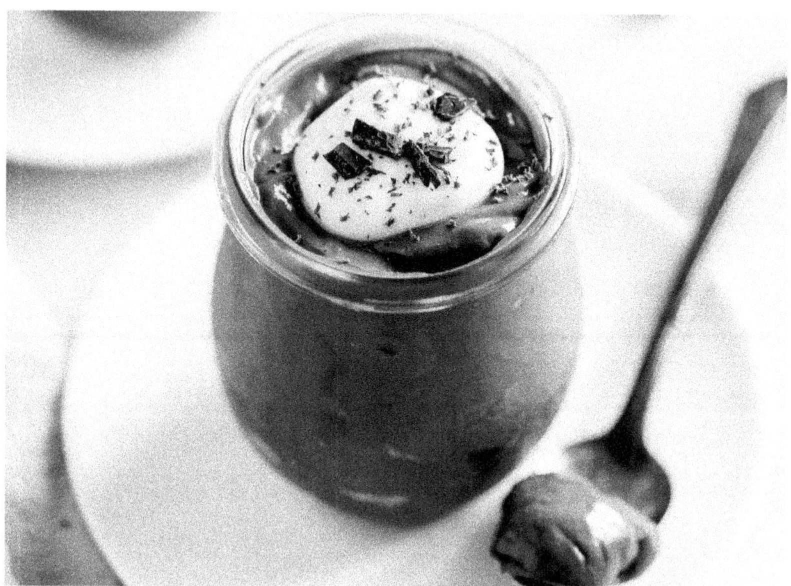

Ingredients

- 2 ripe avocados
- 1/4 cup unsweetened cocoa powder
- 1/4 cup almond milk
- 2 tablespoons maple syrup
- 1 teaspoon vanilla ext

Instructions

1. Blend avocados, cocoa powder, almond milk, maple syrup, and vanilla extract until smooth.
2. Divide into serving cups and refrigerate for at least 2 hours.
3. Garnish with fresh berries or a sprinkle of cocoa before serving.

Nutritional Value

Calories: 180, Healthy Fats: Avocado provides monounsaturated fats.

Brief Description/Backstory

Indulge in a rich and creamy chocolate treat with this sugarless avocado pudding. The avocado adds a velvety texture, while cocoa provides a decadent chocolate flavor.

Berry and Greek Yogurt Parfait

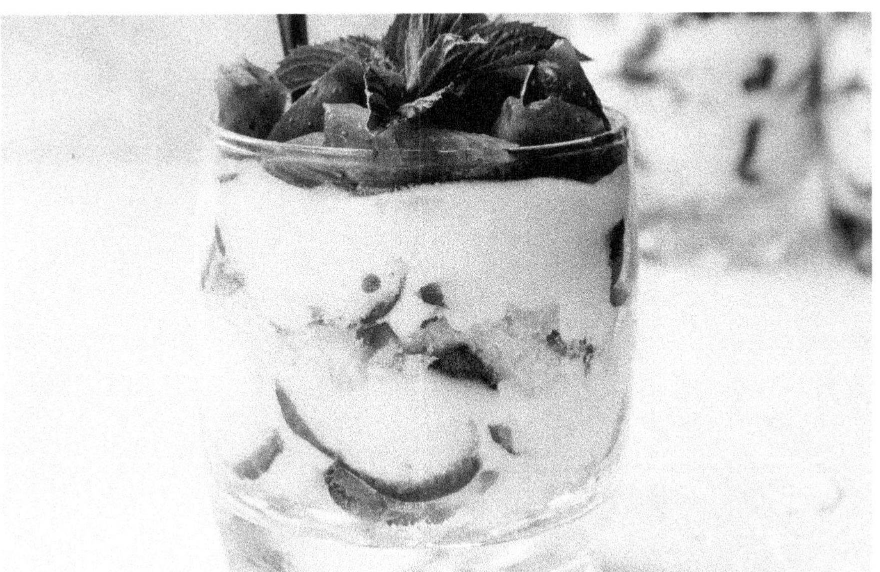

Ingredients

- cups mixed berries (strawberries, blueberries, raspberries)
- 1 cup Greek yogurt
- Drizzle of honey (optional)
- Chopped nuts for crunch

Instructions

1. In glasses or bowls, layer Greek yogurt and mixed berries.
2. Drizzle with honey if desired.
3. Top with chopped nuts for added texture.
4. Enjoy this light and refreshing parfait.

Nutritional Value

Calories: 150, Protein: 12g, Antioxidants: Berries are rich in antioxidants.

Brief Description/Backstory

Create a delightful sugarless dessert with this berry and Greek yogurt parfait. Layers of fresh berries and creamy Greek yogurt offer a guilt-free indulgence.

Coconut Chia Seed Pudding

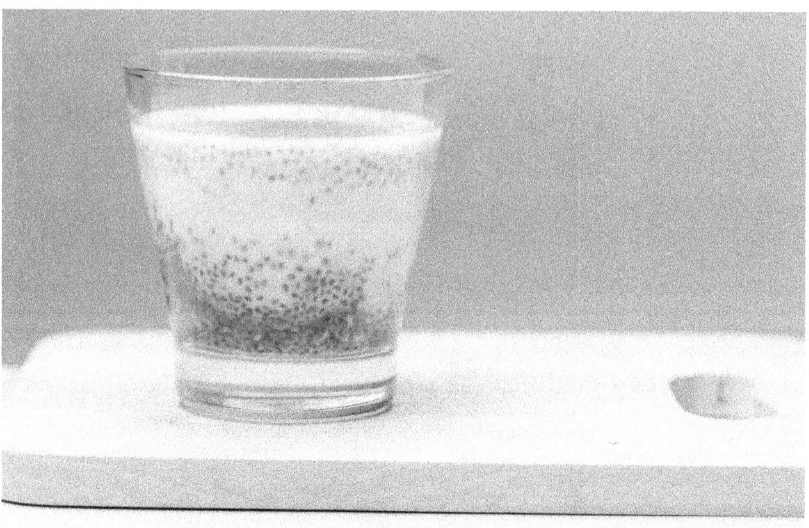

Ingredients

- 1 can coconut milk
- 1/2 cup chia seeds
- 2 tablespoons maple syrup
- 1 teaspoon vanilla extract
- Shredded coconut for garnish

Instructions

1. In a bowl, mix coconut milk, chia seeds, maple syrup, and vanilla extract.
2. Refrigerate for at least 4 hours or overnight.
3. Stir well and divide into serving cups.
4. Garnish with shredded coconut before serving.

Nutritional Value

Calories: 220, Omega-3 Fatty Acids: Chia seeds are rich in omega-3s.

Brief Description/Backstory

Transport yourself to a tropical paradise with this coconut chia seed pudding. A luscious and sugarless dessert that's easy to prepare and full of wholesome ingredients.

Almond Flour Banana Bread

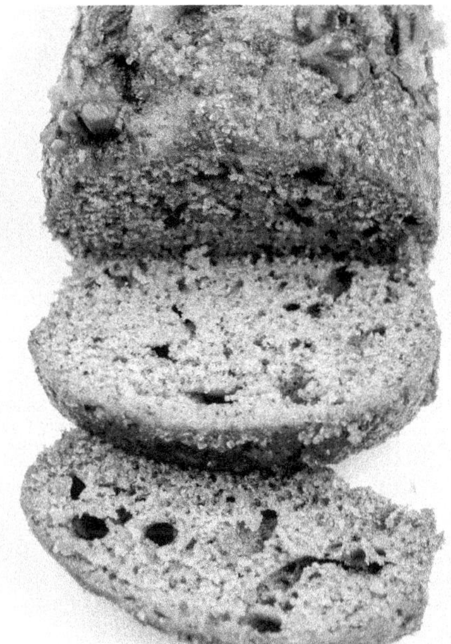

Ingredients

- 2 ripe bananas, mashed
- - 3 eggs
- 1/4 cup coconut oil, melted
- 1 teaspoon vanilla extract
- 2 cups almond flour
- 1 teaspoon baking soda
- Pinch of salt
- Chopped nuts for topping (optional)

Nutritional Value

Calories: 180,
Protein: 6g,
Healthy Fats: Almond flour provides monounsaturated fats.

Instructions

1. Preheat oven to 350°F (175°C). Grease a loaf pan.
2. In a bowl, mix mashed bananas, eggs, melted coconut oil, and vanilla extract.
3. Add almond flour, baking soda, and salt. Stir until combined.
4. Pour batter into the prepared pan, top with chopped nuts if desired.
5. Bake for 45-50 minutes or until a toothpick comes out clean.

Brief Description/Backstory

Satisfy your sweet tooth without added sugars with this almond flour banana bread. Moist, flavorful, and gluten-free, it's a guilt-free dessert indulgence.

Vanilla Chia Seed Pudding with Fresh Fruit

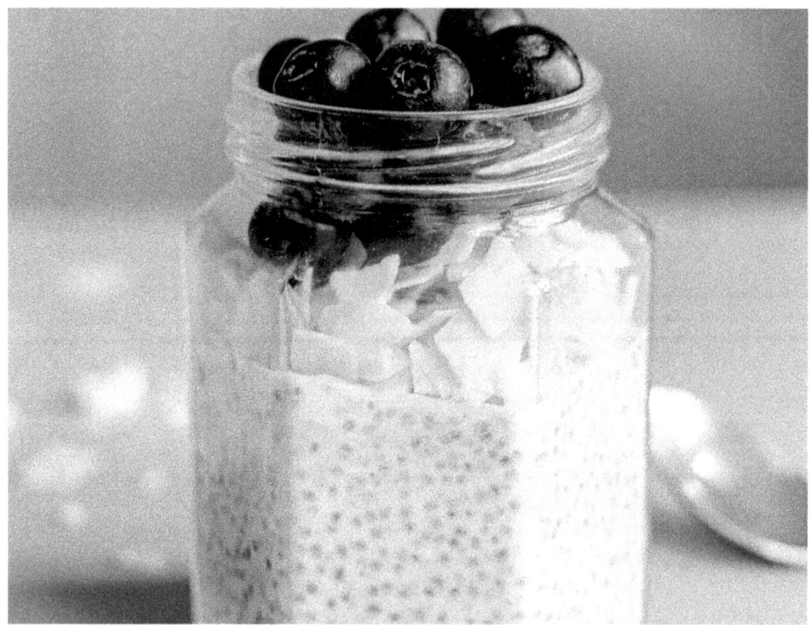

Ingredients

- 1 cup vanilla-flavored almond milk
- 1/2 cup chia seeds
- 1 teaspoon maple syrup (optional)
- 1 teaspoon vanilla extract
- Assorted fresh fruits for topping

Instructions

1. In a bowl, whisk almond milk, chia seeds, maple syrup, and vanilla extract.
2. Refrigerate for at least 2 hours or overnight.
3. Stir well and spoon into serving cups.
4. Top with a variety of fresh fruits before serving.

Brief Description/Backstory

Elevate your dessert experience with this vanilla chia seed pudding topped with a medley of fresh fruits. A delightful and sugarless treat that's as beautiful as it is delicious.

Nutritional Value

Calories: 120, Fiber: 5g.

Baked Apple with Cinnamon and Walnuts

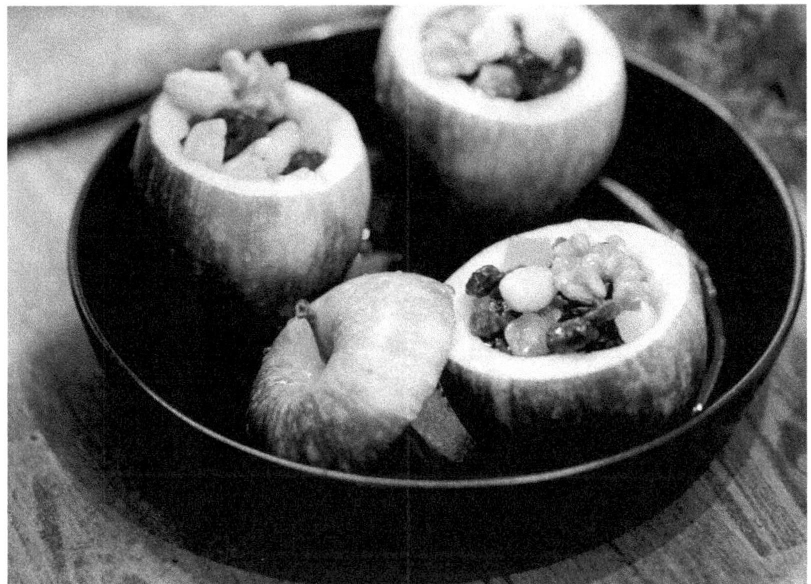

Ingredients

- 2 apples, cored and halved
- 1 teaspoon cinnamon
- 2 tablespoons chopped walnuts
- Drizzle of honey (optional)

Instructions

1. Preheat oven to 375°F (190°C).
2. Place apple halves on a baking sheet.
3. Sprinkle with cinnamon and top with chopped walnuts.
4. Bake for 20-25 minutes or until apples are tender.
5. Drizzle with honey if desired before serving.

Brief Description/Backstory

Experience the warm and comforting flavors of baked apple with cinnamon and walnuts. This sugarless dessert is a wholesome twist on a classic treat.

Nutritional Value

Calories: 150,
Fiber: 6g,
Omega-3 Fatty Acids: Walnuts provide omega-3s.

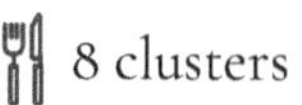 8 clusters

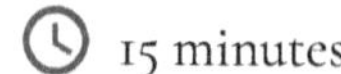 15 minutes

Dark Chocolate and Almond Clusters

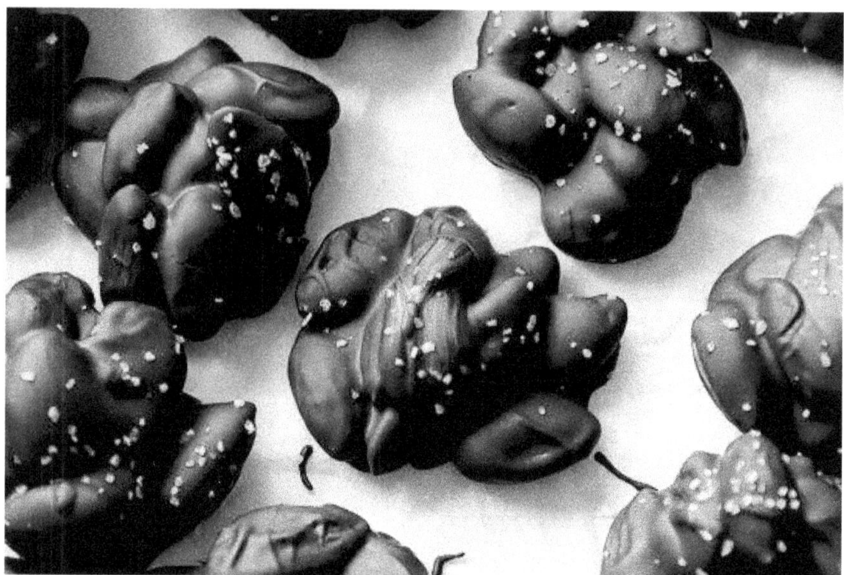

Ingredients

- cup dark chocolate chips (70% cocoa or higher)
- 1 cup almonds, roughly chopped
- Sea salt for sprinkling

Instructions

1. Melt dark chocolate in a heatproof bowl over simmering water or in the microwave.
2. Stir in chopped almonds until well coated.
3. Spoon clusters onto a parchment-lined tray.
4. Sprinkle with sea salt and let them cool until chocolate hardens.

Nutritional Value

Calories: 90,
Healthy Fats:
Almonds provide
monounsaturated fats.

Brief Description/Backstory

Satisfy your chocolate cravings with these dark chocolate and almond clusters. A sugarless indulgence that combines the richness of dark chocolate with the crunch of almonds.

Lemon Blueberry Cheesecake Bites

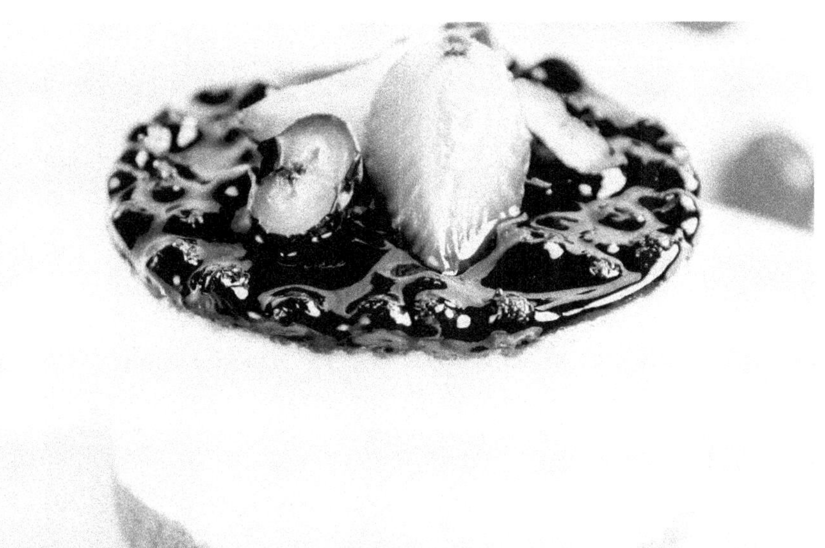

Ingredients

- 1 cup cream cheese, softened
- 1/4 cup Greek yogurt
- Zest and juice of 1 lemon
- 2 tablespoons powdered erythritol (or sweetener of choice)
- Fresh blueberries for topping

Nutritional Value

Calories: 70,
Protein: 3g.

Instructions

1. In a bowl, beat cream cheese, Greek yogurt, lemon zest, lemon juice, and sweetener until smooth.
2. Spoon mixture into mini muffin cups.
3. Chill in the refrigerator for at least 2 hours.
4. Top with fresh blueberries before serving.

Brief Description/Backstory

Delight your taste buds with these lemon blueberry cheesecake bites. A sugarless and bite-sized version of the classic dessert that's bursting with fruity flavors.

Pumpkin Spice Chia Seed Pudding

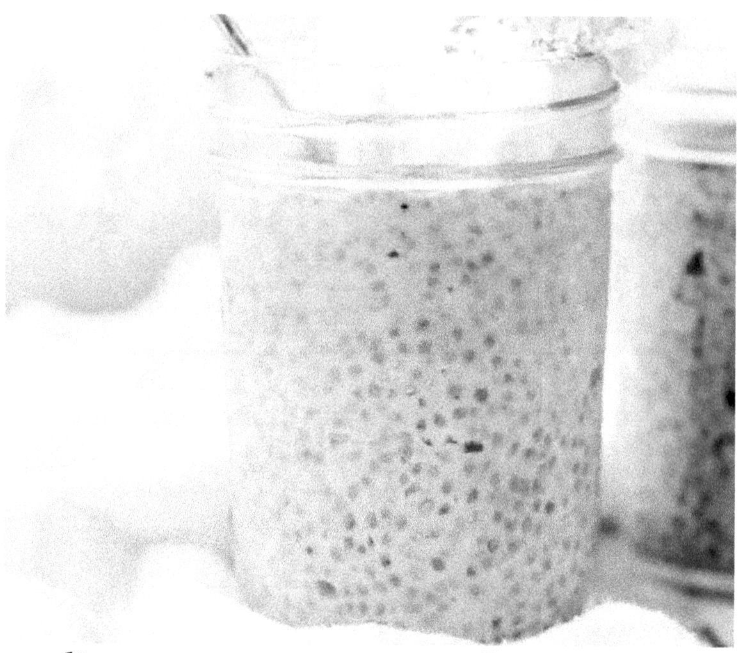

Ingredients

- 1 cup pumpkin puree
- 2 cups unsweetened almond milk
- 1/2 cup chia seeds
- 2 tablespoons maple syrup (optional)
- 1 teaspoon pumpkin spice blend

Nutritional Value

Calories: 160,
Fiber: 8g.

Instructions

1. In a bowl, combine diced tomatoes, fresh basil, and minced garlic.
2. Drizzle with balsamic vinegar and toss gently.
3. Toast baguette slices and top with the tomato basil mixture.
4. Serve your delightful tomato basil bruschetta.

Brief Description/Backstory

Celebrate the flavors of fall with this pumpkin spice chia seed pudding. A sugarless dessert that combines the warmth of pumpkin spice with the nutritional benefits of chia seeds.

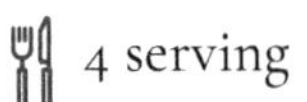

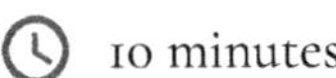

Mango Coconut Nice Cream

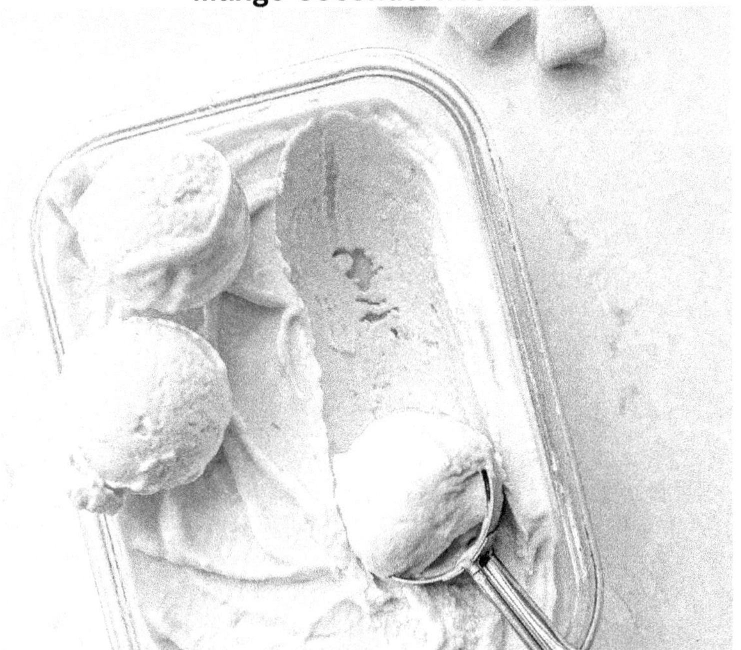

Ingredients

- 2 cups frozen mango chunks
- 1 can coconut milk (full fat)
- 1 teaspoon vanilla extract
- Unsweetened coconut flakes for topping

Instructions

1. In a blender, combine frozen mango, coconut milk, and vanilla extract.
2. Blend until smooth and creamy.
3. Transfer to a container and freeze for at least 4 hours.
4. Scoop and top with unsweetened coconut flakes before serving.

Brief Description/Backstory

Experience the tropical bliss of mango coconut nice cream. This sugarless frozen dessert is a guilt-free alternative to traditional ice cream, blending the sweetness of mango with creamy coconut.

Nutritional Value

Calories: 120, Healthy Fats: Coconut milk provides healthy fats.

QUIZ TIME!

How often do you experience intense cravings for sugary foods or drinks?

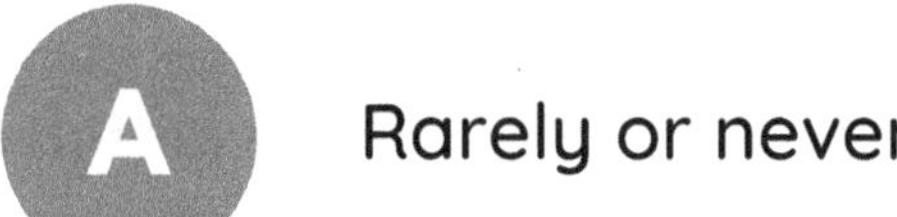

Rarely or never

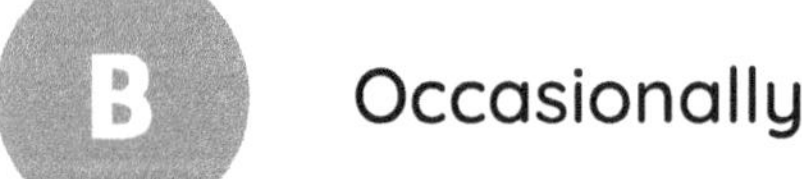

Occasionally

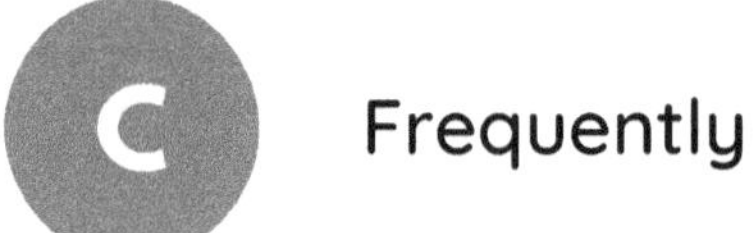

Frequently

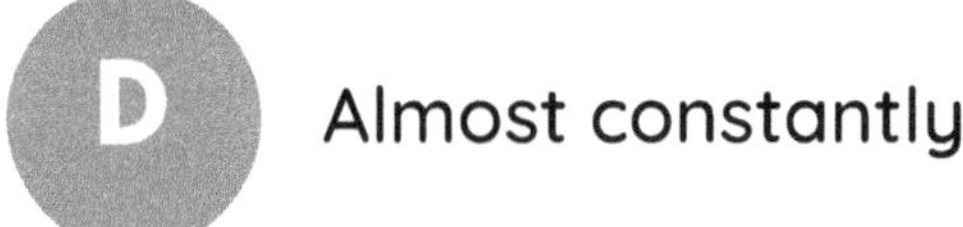

Almost constantly

QUIZ TIME!

How much added sugar do you estimate you consume on a daily basis?

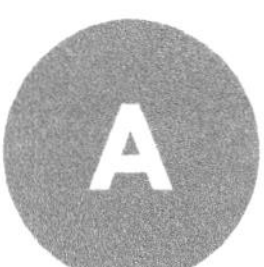

Minimal or none

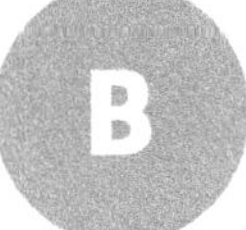

Some, but within recommended guidelines

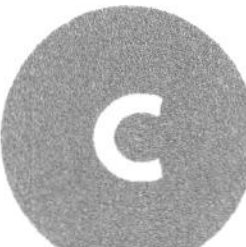

Exceeds recommended guidelines

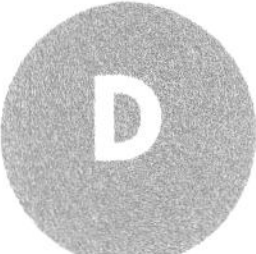

Excessive; I'm unsure of the quantity

QUIZ TIME!

Do you often turn to sugary foods or drinks as a source of comfort during stressful or emotional situations?

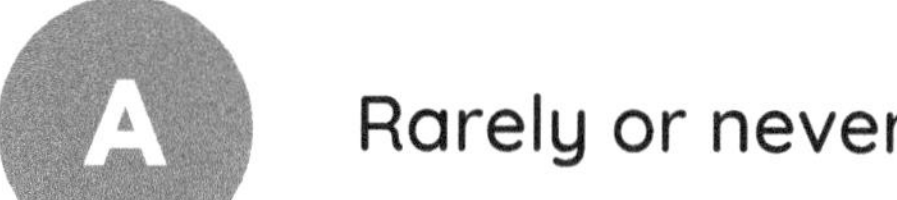

A Rarely or never

B Occasionally

C Frequently

D Almost always

QUIZ TIME!

How do you feel when you attempt to cut back on sugar consumption?

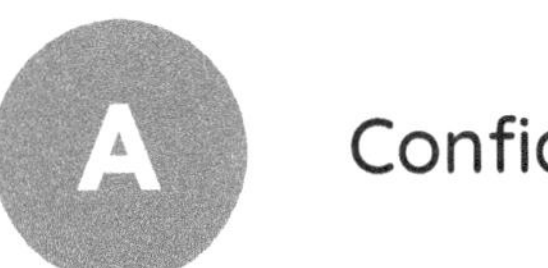

Confident and in control

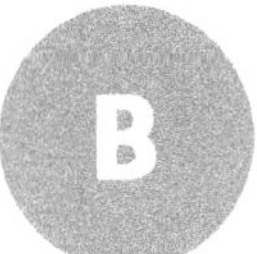

Somewhat challenged, but manageable

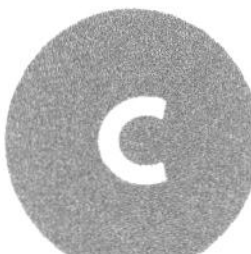

Anxious or irritable

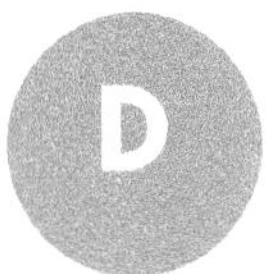

Overwhelmed or defeated

QUIZ TIME!

Do you find yourself hiding or sneaking sugary snacks or drinks?

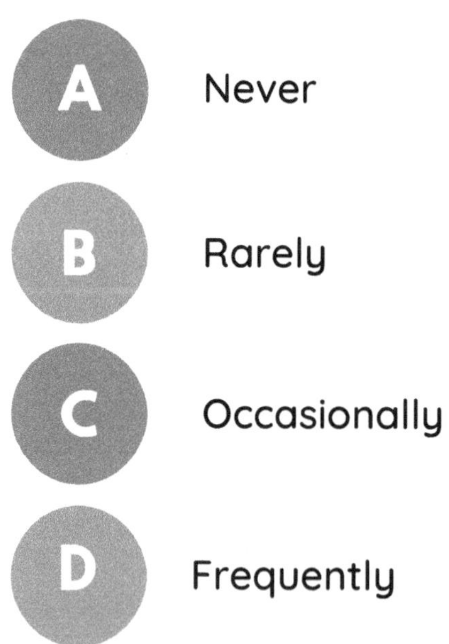

A Never

B Rarely

C Occasionally

D Frequently

QUIZ TIME !

Have you tried to reduce your sugar intake in the past, only to find it challenging or unsuccessful?

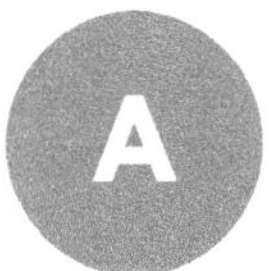

No, I've never tried

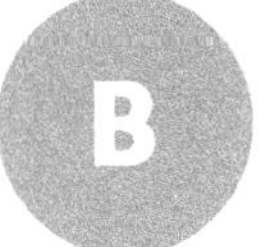

Yes, but with moderate success

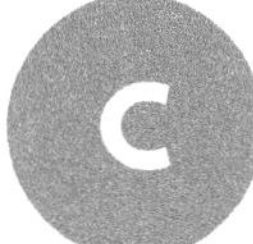

Yes, and it was difficult

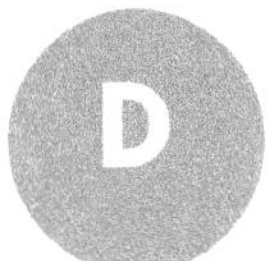

Yes, and I was unsuccessful

QUIZ TIME!

Each question carries a score based on your response. Assign the following values

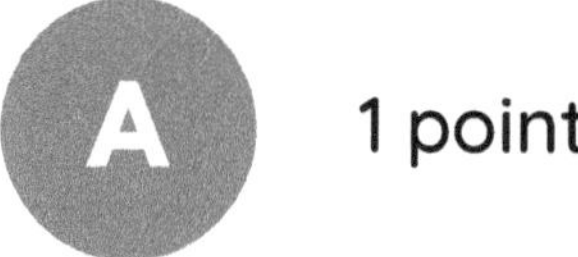

1 point

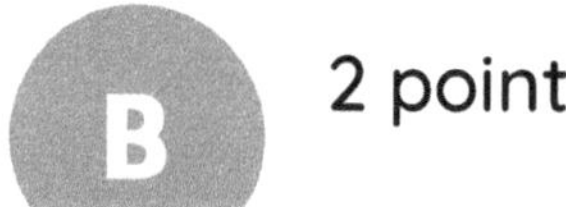

2 point

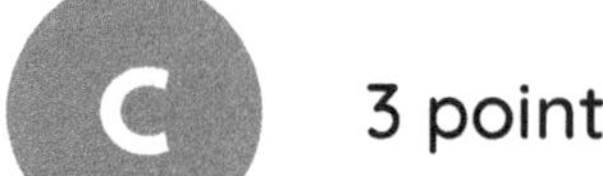

3 point

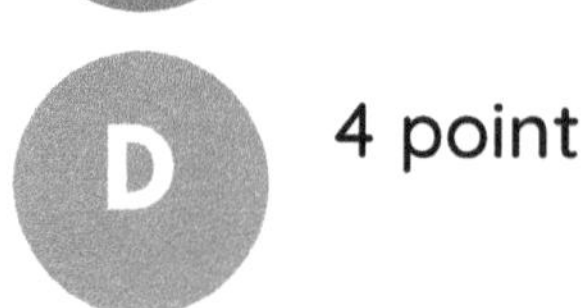

4 point

Interpretation

6-10 points: Low likelihood of sugar addiction
11-15 points: Moderate risk; consider evaluating and adjusting your sugar consumption
16-20 points: Elevated risk; your relationship with sugar may be impacting your well-being
21-24 points: High risk; seek professional guidance to address potential sugar addiction

Understanding Your Results

Low Likelihood of Sugar Addiction (6-10 points)
Congratulations! Your quiz results suggest a low likelihood of sugar addiction. You likely have a healthy relationship with sugar, incorporating it into your diet without dependency. Continue making mindful choices to maintain your balanced approach.

Moderate Risk (11-15 points)
Your results indicate a moderate risk of sugar addiction. Consider evaluating your sugar consumption patterns and exploring ways to reduce your intake. Adopting mindful eating practices and seeking support can contribute to healthier habits.

Elevated Risk (16-20 points)
An elevated risk suggests that your relationship with sugar may be impacting your well-being. Assess your consumption patterns, identify triggers, and consider implementing strategies to reduce sugar intake. Seeking guidance from a nutritionist or healthcare professional may be beneficial.

High Risk (21-24 points)
Your results indicate a high risk of sugar addiction. It's crucial to address this issue for your overall health. Seek professional guidance, consider counseling or support groups, and work towards implementing sustainable changes in your diet and lifestyle.

CONCLUSION

Embracing a Sugarless Lifestyle

As you reach the conclusion of your journey towards a sugarless lifestyle, it's essential to take a moment to reflect on the transformative path you've undertaken. The decision to reduce and eliminate added sugars from your diet is a commendable commitment to your overall health and well-being. In this closing chapter, we'll explore the significance of reflecting on your journey, celebrating successes, and embracing a sugarless future.

Reflecting on Your Journey

As you look back on the chapters of this transformative experience, consider the strides you've made in understanding the impact of sugar on your health. The knowledge gained about the hidden sources of sugar, the addictive nature of this sweet substance, and the practical steps to break free from its grasp is an empowering foundation for a healthier lifestyle.

Reflection allows you to acknowledge the hurdles you faced and the strength you discovered within yourself to overcome them. Take a moment to appreciate the progress made, no matter how small, as each step contributes to the larger journey towards improved health.

Celebrating Successes
Amidst the challenges and adjustments, it's crucial to celebrate your successes along the way. Whether it's overcoming sugar cravings, adopting new and nourishing habits, or experiencing positive changes in your overall well-being, these achievements deserve recognition.

Consider keeping a journal of your successes, no matter how modest they may seem. Recognizing and celebrating these milestones not only reinforces positive behavior but also serves as a source of motivation for the continued pursuit of a sugarless lifestyle.

Embracing a Sugarless Future
As you stand at the threshold of the future, envision the possibilities that await you in a sugarless life. Embrace the long-term success that comes with nurturing a healthier relationship with food and making conscious choices. The journey doesn't end with the last page of this book; it's an ongoing narrative that you have the power to shape.

Continue exploring new recipes, refining your coping mechanisms for stress and setbacks, and staying connected with a community that shares your commitment to a sugar-free existence. Remember, this lifestyle is not about deprivation but about abundance—a wealth of health, vitality, and the joy of savoring natural flavors.

In the pursuit of a sugarless future, prioritize self-care, mindfulness, and a holistic approach to well-being. Surround yourself with positivity, stay attuned to your body's signals, and relish the sense of freedom that comes with breaking free from the shackles of excessive sugar consumption.

Closing Thoughts
In concluding this guide, let the closing thoughts be a reminder that your journey towards a sugarless lifestyle is a continuous narrative of self-discovery and empowerment. You are not just eliminating sugar; you are rewriting the story of your health, one chapter at a time.

As you turn the final pages of this book, carry forward the knowledge, resilience, and determination you've gained. Your commitment to a sugarless lifestyle is an investment in your present and future well-being, a gift that keeps on giving with every healthy choice you make.

May your path be filled with vibrant health, culinary delights, and the satisfaction of embracing a sugarless future—one that reflects your dedication to a life well-lived.